What about me?

Finding SELF-LOVE through SELF-CARE

What about me?

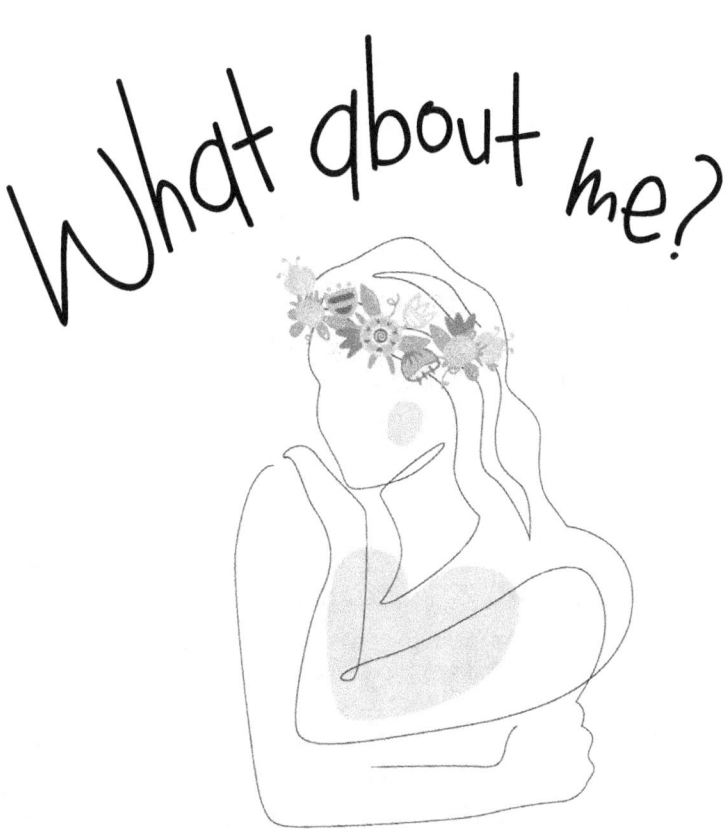

Finding **SELF-LOVE** through **SELF-CARE**

CHRISSY KOHUT

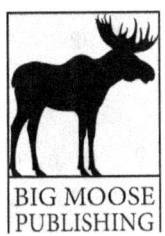

BIG MOOSE
PUBLISHING

ISBN: 978-1-989840-76-4 (sc)
ISBN: 978-1-989840-77-1 (ebook)

Big Moose Publishing 10/2024

*For Mom, the dancing queen, who not only brought my soul to life,
but also taught me the importance of self-care and self-love.
I love and miss you dearly. XO*

Contents

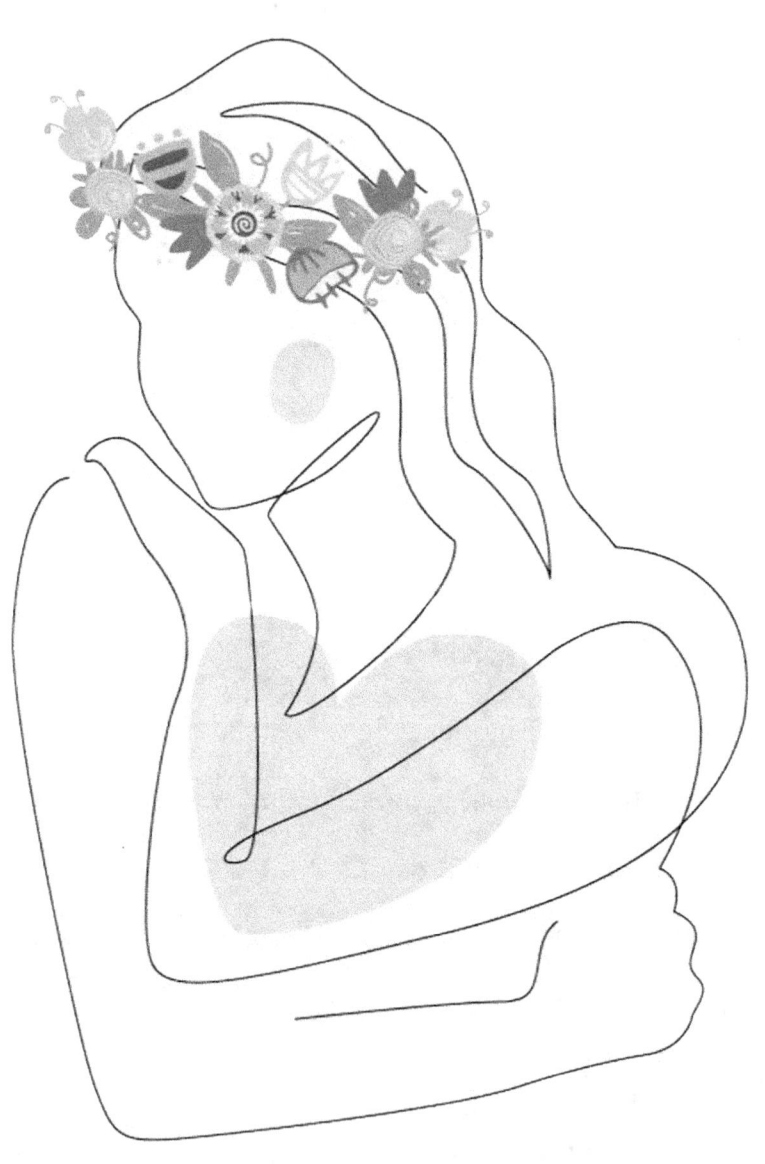

Introduction

"What about me?"

I can remember muttering those words so many times when I was a young mom and young wife. So many days and nights I spent catering to little humans, and to my husband, making sure all their wants and needs were met. If I am going to be honest, I muttered those words, *What About Me?* pretty much most of my life.

Any other people pleasers out there? I wasn't taught while growing up in the 70s and 80s to ask for what I wanted so I sure as hell never asked for what I needed. In my generation as a female, you were taught through the actions of older generations and the media that your role as a female was to worry about everyone BUT yourself. If you did dare to worry about yourself then you were deemed selfish. So naturally, when I became a mother and wife, my focus was to take care of them. And like most young moms and wives, I dove head first always trying to make my husband and my kids happy, even if that meant I put my happiness to the side. Don't get me wrong, making my kids and husband happy makes me very happy. Watching them smile and laugh and fulfill their dreams lights up my heart. But here's the thing: if you are always pouring yourself into someone else without refilling yourself, eventually you run out of something to pour. When you are empty, you have nothing left to give to anyone, let alone yourself.

I never learned to express my wants and needs. I never learned to use my voice. I would keep all my emotions bottled up inside. Don't worry. My emotions would come out eventually, like a tornado storm, typically in the form of stomping my feet or slamming cabinet doors (thanks for teaching me how to slam a cabinet door mom, LOL) or screaming while tears ran down my face saying things in the moment that I wouldn't remember later, because I was so far gone in my swirling of my emotions I had no idea what I was thinking let alone saying. Sound familiar?

This is what happens when you don't put your wants or needs first, ever. You become resentful. You become depressed. You feel invisible. You feel unworthy. And you get angry. Very, very angry. Then, one day you cannot take it anymore and you explode, and along comes the tornado. You are cursing out your husband. You are screaming at your kids. You go off on a tangent at your best friend. You even get snarky with your dog. Once the winds of your emotions end you are left with your husband, or kids, or friend, or dog looking at you with their head cocked to one side bewildered at what just transpired. Most likely your husband will ask you if you are about to get your period. Then you will run off crying hysterically all the while thinking nobody cares about you. Still sound familiar?

Let me set something straight. The people in your day-to-day life, even the dog, care about you. They may piss you off from time to time and do some stupid shit. There will be times you have every right to be angry and disagree with them. They may very well be the cause of a small breeze at the beginning of your storm, but you, my friend, are the reason the trees were lifted and your house was shredded. Instead of gently grounding yourself in the moment of the breeze, you allowed yourself to be picked up and carried away. Like I said, the people in your life, they care about you. But you, you don't.

Once the hysterical sobbing stops, the tears dry up, and the pounding headache from crying sets in, you begin to whisper to yourself, "What about me?" Those words, my friend, are not your soul crying out for someone to love you. Those words are your soul crying out for you to love yourself again. Those words mean you need to return home; and the only way home is through self-love. The way to self-love is by creating a daily self-care practice filled with habits and rituals throughout the day that fill you up with love.

If what I am saying is resonating with you even in the slightest way, then my friend, I wrote this book just for you. I wish I had known earlier in my life how important it is to love myself first before I loved anyone else, even my kids. I wish someone would have sat me down and looked me in the eyes and told me that the key to a healthy and happy life is self-love. That nobody and no thing can make me happy except me. That making other people happy is an act of love not an act of duty.

As a society we have become so far removed from loving ourselves. Between the expectations of our family of origin, our partners, our children, our education, our life experiences, our childhood trauma, our religion, and don't forget social media, we have forgotten that our birthright is self-love. So, as you read these pages, I want you to know my words are my eyes looking into yours telling you that your path to self-love is taking care of yourself daily: mind, body, and spirit; and I am here to guide you to your path of self-love through self-care.

By the end of this book I want you and anyone else reading this to be me-ish. Oh, what's me-ish? I will be happy to share that information with you.

Me-ish is when you take time for yourself daily and fill your cup up with as much love and affection as you do others. When we are me-ish, we are not disregarding our responsibilities such as home, family, friends, and work. On the contrary we are more attentive and present to our responsibilities because we have taken the time to also take care of ourselves and fill our cup allowing an overflow of abundance of ourselves to give to others.

I want you, my friend, to wake up every morning feeling a little me-ish and with this thought, "It's a good day to have a good day," because you are armed with a toolbox filled with self-care tools.

CHAPTER ONE

What Is Self-Care?

Self-care is a trendy word these days. Seems like everyone is using it. Yet the word is so vaguely used that nobody is quite sure what it is, what it means, and the question then becomes, *"How does one self-care?"*

I have been studying and practicing self-care for over thirty years. In those thirty years I have found that self-care is about taking care of the whole self: mind, body, and spirit, daily. Yes, I said DAILY. You can do all the crunches and eat the greens, but if your head (mind) and heart (spirit) aren't aligned with your body, then you never truly are healthy and happy. Thus, living the life of your dreams can be difficult to obtain.

What I have also come to find is that when our mind, body, and spirit are aligned, we are practicing self-love. I have seen family, friends, and clients countlessly focus on one area of themselves, assuming if they get that part just right, everything in life will fall into place. It is like trying to watch someone build a home with only one wall up. You need a strong foundation, a sturdy floor with four walls, to build a home. Eventually, you add the roof. But the roof is always temporary because as long as that foundation is strong you can raise that roof as high to the sky as you want.

The same goes for yourself. You need a strong foundation for warmth, comfort, and protection. A foundation where you can be free, creative, and loved for your authentic self. Your daily self-care practice is your foundation for your home filled with self-love.

Over the last thirty years I have created habits and rituals focusing on my physical, emotional, social, intellectual, and spiritual self. These five areas are the areas of self that I find most crucial to focus on daily to keep my mind, body, and spirit aligned. When these five areas are aligned and centered, most days life just flows beautifully. Notice I said most days. This is because even though I practice daily self-care, there are things in my life I can't control, even through self-care. There are so many external things that are out of my control. When those external things begin to brew like a storm about to wreak havoc on my home, meaning myself, that is when I use my foundation. I shut the doors and lock them, close the windows and blinds, and seek shelter within. I pull out the tools from my toolbox and I work to keep myself safe, comforted, and warm. But most of all, I work to make sure I am loved by me.

Loving yourself is very important. I had the best teacher in the world to teach me that lesson, my mom. However, her lesson was heartbreaking. My mom didn't have the best childhood. She was one of the oldest of nine kids. My grandfather was a disabled veteran from WWII. When his army tank was hit by a missile, he was the only one to survive. However, he survived with severe burns that left him with no face or ears for that matter. He spent years in VA hospitals growing skin grafts so that the doctors could perform reconstructive surgery to build him a new face and give him back some ears. Back then plastic surgery wasn't what it is today, and back then people who looked deformed had a very difficult time finding employment. So, my mom grew up in the projects with a very angry and violent father who drank a lot.

My mother married my father at the age of 19 and, as most women do, they marry men who resemble their father in personality. My dad isn't an angry or violent man, but he did drink a lot. Shortly after my parents were married, my sister and I were born. Oh, did I mention I was a twin? Imagine having your wants and needs met when you are twins. You don't have to imagine; I will tell you. It isn't easy. Don't get me wrong. I know my parents loved me, but I have been suppressing my wants and needs since the womb.

When my sister and I were born my mom had an emergency C-section. She was two weeks overdue and had toxemia. My sister and I were removed from her belly and, shortly after, my mom had a grand seizure and went into a coma. The coma didn't last long, and eventually my mom and my sister and I were released from the hospital.

My dad says even to this day how my mom was amazing with me and my sister. He wasn't home a lot to help with my sister and me, because he was always juggling two or three jobs. But he would come home and the house was always clean, food was always prepared, and my sister and I were well taken care of.

My mom was that way most of my life. She took pride in our home and her appearance. She had the most beautiful finger nails that were always perfectly filed and painted. Her hair was always perfect and she never really wore makeup around the house, but when she went somewhere she was always put together. But honestly, she didn't need the makeup. She was just naturally beautiful.

Growing up my mom and I would argue because I was the complete opposite of her as a child. As an adult I became more like her, especially with my home. My appearance, not so much, but I digress. I think the thing that drove her nuts the most was that my clothes were always wrinkly. I didn't care, but she sure as hell did. She would constantly make comments about how wrinkly my clothes were. That was my mom though. When she thought something about you then you knew it, but she never let us know what she thought of herself.

My mom was also known for her decorating abilities. Honestly, she should have been an interior designer, or maybe she was in a previous life. Anyone and everyone who entered our home would walk around taking notice of the decor in our home making wonderful comments. My mom knew how to make a house a home. She also knew how to make you feel welcome in our home, so much so that we often had family members living with us when times were tough for them. That was my mom, always taking care of everyone. That was, everyone but herself.

My parents divorced when I was in my early twenties, shortly after I had my first born child. It wasn't a surprise to my sister and me, or really anyone, that my parents got divorced. My parents undoubtedly loved one another, but they loved one another like best friends. They had been through a lot together, but being together, well that wasn't the best scenario for the two of them. I am grateful that they remained friends through the years though. I imagine at times that had to be hard. But then again, that was my mom, always pushing her feelings aside so everyone else would be happy.

When my mom was in her forties she was diagnosed with type 2 diabetes and, as the years went on, her doctor would beg and plead with her to take care of herself and the diabetes. He was so concerned that when my dad would have an appointment, he would mention to my dad his concerns for my mom. Years went on and slowly I started to notice subtle changes in my mom. One summer my husband and I were throwing our annual 4th of July party with our family and friends. My mom showed up and when she walked in the door, I was taken back by the way she looked. At that time my mom lived a significant amount of time away from my house, so I didn't see her as often when she still lived in our home town. Her hair was done, but she didn't have any makeup on, which was odd because she always showed up at a party with at least a little bit of makeup on. What was most concerning was her nails were long, not filed, and not painted. I shook it off and thought maybe I was overreacting.

Later that day my dad pulled me aside and asked me what was going on with my mom. His words were, "Did you see her fingernails?! They aren't painted." That was the beginning of a very long and painful journey with my mom and her health.

My mom eventually wound up in the hospital with congestive heart failure. The cause of the congestive heart failure was due to kidney failure. The cause of the kidney failure was due to not taking care of her type 2 diabetes. I spent the following years in and out of dialysis centers, emergency rooms, hospital rooms, and rehab facilities. My mom suffered from a heart attack, a stroke, and multiple broken bones because she became so weak from being filled with fluid. She would miss multiple rounds of dialysis, then she would fall and break a bone.

This was her pattern. She would be released from the hospital after almost succumbing to death and then be very mindful of taking care of herself for a while. Then slowly, she would start slipping into the routine of just not giving a fuck. She would eat the wrong foods, and smoke cigarettes while still being hooked to her oxygen machine. The worst though was she would skip dialysis. I mean I can't even imagine what kind of toll it takes on a person to be stuck to a machine three days a week for hours, as your blood is being removed and then put back into your body. It has to be emotionally and physically exhausting.

Every time she skipped dialysis though, it would take weeks off of her life. Not minutes, not days, weeks. And she skipped dialysis A LOT. The times she would skip we would beg and plead and cry and scream for her to go. But she would tell us to fuck off and then just stare off into the distance.

Later during my therapy sessions, I would learn that staring off in the distance was her disassociating so that she didn't have to deal with the trauma she was feeling. The last four years of my mom's life were horrible. The last two years, well they were fucking horrific. My sister and I dubbed her "The Medical Marvel" because the doctors would look at her chart and then stare up at us and say, "After reading your mother's chart I don't understand how she's even still here with us."

For the last four years of her life, the woman I knew, who raised me, who was always put together, no longer existed. I often say I lost my mom four years before she actually transitioned over to the other side, because the woman who existed in those last four years of her life was not my mom.

This woman wore hideous wigs, because she didn't want to do her hair. She would never wear makeup. She barely got dressed out of her pajamas. She wouldn't cook or clean. Hell, it was a fight to get her to shower. I missed her smelling of soap and perfume. My mom always used to smell good. Not those last four years though. She just sat around watching the same movies over and over and over again like Pearl Harbor or the Hallmark Channel. Literally, I would have to confirm with rehabs what cable service they received so that she could watch the Hallmark Channel when she had a stay at a rehab, or she was adamant she wasn't going there. She was still feisty. I will give her that.

In the spring of 2019, my mom suffered a stroke. It took some time and physically she bounced back pretty well, but cognitively she was beginning to really slip away. Then in the fall of 2019, she fell and broke her femur bone. She survived the surgery, and when they wheeled her into the room the doctor pulled me out into the hallway. Typically, when you are at a hospital, the doctors and nurses see so many patients they don't remember who you are after you leave. Not me. My mom was such a frequent flier at the local hospitals that we all knew each other when we saw each other coming down the hallway. I'll never forget the doctor's words after my mom's surgery. "This break is your mom's tipping point. A tipping point is where it can no longer get better. It will only be downhill with her from here. Typically, when someone as fragile as she is sustains a break like this, they may have a year left."

You would think that I would have been upset over what he had just said to me, but I wasn't. I wasn't, because I knew he was right. I knew in my gut that what was to come was going to be worse than my family could imagine. The vision of my son sitting next to my mom in the ER months later, holding her hand crying to her that it is okay to let go, while she had a BIPAP mask over her mouth pumping oxygen into her so that she could breathe, as she laid there unconscious is a vision I will never be able to remove from my memory. Or standing in the doorway of the ER as they were trying to wheel in the dialysis machine, and her oxygen tanked, so then the doctor came flying in pushing the nurses out of the way and proceeded to punch my mom with her fist in her chest to bring her back. The Medical Marvel survived again. Or the times trying to hold her up and put her on the portable toilet next to bed, and as I placed her down on the seat she would pass out and fall backwards, and I would have to catch her.

To this day my sister and I are so triggered at the sound of an ambulance that we text one another when we see or hear one. For me, every time my phone rings I have an immediate panic response that something is wrong and any time my phone lights up with a text around 11:00 p.m., I have to take a deep inhale and exhale before reading the text, because my mom was notorious for night time ER trips. To this day, even though my mom has been gone for a few years now, my purse is always packed as if I am going to be spending hours in a waiting room with a phone charger, snacks, and water.

A year after my mom broke her femur, she was admitted into hospice. A week later, she took her last breath. All the people who meant the most to her came to visit her. Those who couldn't make it, because we still were in the midst of a pandemic, Face Timed with her. In true fashion, my mom rallied for a week. She was admitted on a Friday and by Sunday night she was quickly deteriorating. Monday morning she was wide awake. The nurses said patients sometimes do this. They call it "their last hoorah". So, we brought her all her favorites, McDonalds, coffee, donuts, and her dog, Stella. The Medical Marvel decided to hoorah so long she almost got kicked out of the hospice facility and sent home on hospice. Health insurance companies are so fucked up! However, mom began to decline and passed peacefully with myself and my sister by her side. I think it was fitting that she was there for our first breath and we were there for her last.

As we stood there looking at her finally free of pain and suffering, we both agreed we felt such relief in knowing she wasn't suffering. That was when I realized that although my mom's death certificate would state renal kidney failure, what my mom died of was a broken heart. Not a broken heart because of someone else, but a broken heart because she didn't love herself enough to take care of herself. A broken heart that was trying to fill voids by pleasing other people and trying to find happiness externally. I truly believe my mom's death could have been prevented solely by self-love.

I don't want to become my mom. At least not in that way, and I don't want you to become my mom either. No one deserves to suffer like that. And no one deserves to watch someone they love suffer that way either. I am so god damn grateful that in the midst of all that was so very fucked up over the last four years of my mom's life, I realized my mom's purpose on this earth and her purpose in regards to my life. Her purpose wasn't to put me through pain and suffering as I watched her in pain and suffering. It was to teach me all the ways I should and shouldn't treat myself, and even better yet, let others treat me, so in turn I can teach you.

She also taught me that life is so very short. My mom died at a young 69 years old. I had just turned 50 years old when she passed away. If I followed her path of not practicing daily self-care, I would have only had another 19 years left of my life. I don't want to only live 19 more years. I still have shit to do, things to see, and people to meet in my life. Most of all, I NEVER want my children to have to suffer through what I did, watching my mom suffer, especially in those last four years.

I understand we have no control over disease, sometimes it just happens, but my mom's disease was preventable. If she had just taken better care of herself, I truly believe that she would still be here. She would have seen my two grandsons, her great grandchildren, being born. She would have been at my oldest daughter's wedding. She would have seen my youngest daughter graduate with her Master's degree and become a therapist. She should still be here, but she's not, and I will be damned if I miss out on life, because I am so comfortable in my discomfort that I won't take care of myself.

I am not doing it for just my kids and my husband. I am doing it for me. Because I deserve to live a healthy and happy life. And god damn it, so do you!

I want you to truly pay attention to what I am about to say, because I do believe this is one of the main root causes of why most people do not take care of themselves. Self-care is not selfish! Let me say it again. SELF-CARE IS NOT SELFISH! Taking care of yourself and making sure that you are healthy and happy is not selfish. It is extremely important and extremely necessary. My mom taught me what NOT to do to live a healthy and happy life. She chose not to take care of herself. She allowed other people's wants and needs to always come before hers. She thought that happiness was within other people instead of within herself. That is not the example I want to be for my kids. I want to lead as an example of what TO DO to live a healthy and happy life for my kids. I want to take care of myself; mind, body, and spirit. I want to be there for the people I love and cherish the most, but also for myself. I want to know that if I am ever alone in the world, I am still happy, because my happiness is inside me not dependent on something outside of me.

Happiness is not in the validation that I'm the best mom or wife or daughter or sister or friend. It's in knowing I am the best version of me that I can be according to me. When we are kind and compassionate and giving to ourselves, we are the best version of ourselves. Sure, being there for other people can make you feel happy, but what percentage of yourself are you giving to other people when you are depleted? Wouldn't you rather be able to give 100% of yourself to the people you love, because you are capable, because you took the time to take care of yourself? Or would you rather be giving 50% of yourself, because you are so burnt out and tired or sick, because you didn't take the time to care for you? We are of no service to others unless we are of service to ourselves first.

I am going to give you a hard truth. You are more important to you than anyone else. I would always say to my husband that "at the end of the day when you put your head on your pillow you only have yourself". Man, he would get so pissed off at me, because he didn't understand the true meaning of what I was saying. He gets it now, but he thought I meant that I felt I had nobody in my life that loved me or that I could lean on.

On the contrary, I know I am loved and I have my tribe of people I can lean onto in good times and in bad. But the reality is that we live so many seasons of life, and in those seasons people will come and go. Some will leave voluntarily. Some you will let go for various reasons. Most tragically, some people will leave us when they pass on and leave this earth. When we put so much validation of our happiness into one of those people, when they do leave us, we have no idea how to move forward in life without them. We become stuck, depressed, angry, sick, and lost. When you know that at the end of the day you always have yourself, you will learn not to become stuck, depressed, angry, sick or lost when you lose someone or something.

Of course, you will feel the emotions and ride the waves of grief while mourning those relationships. But you will walk away with the love and the valuable lessons they were meant to give you from their presence in your life. Each person we encounter, whether it was for a few minutes or a few years, was destined to be placed there for a reason. So, you see it's not selfish to take care of yourself and love yourself. It is important to take care of yourself, because you need you. There is no guarantee that the people you love will always be there. I know it sounds fucked up, but it is the truth.

The happiness and love you receive from other people is just an extra plus in life. It's like the sprinkles to your ice cream cone. You HAVE to find happiness and love within yourself and be okay with that, because sometimes there might not be any sprinkles left for your ice cream cone.

Your kids not only hear every word you speak, but they watch every move you make. I did it with my mom and my kids did it with me. My kids are now in their twenties and I am watching them not only make positive changes in their lives, because of things they have heard me say and things they have seen me do, but I also see them making some of the same mistakes. You will most likely see your kids do the same.

We are only human and we are products of the environment we grew up in. Whatever shit storm you grew up with, you will be damn sure to bring that pile with you when raising your own children. You most likely will repeat the habits or you'll be so hell bent not to be anything like your parent(s) that you will go to the extremes to be the polar opposite of how they raised you. That approach too, typically brings its own pile of issues.

Through my self-care practice I can look back with awareness now at the times I did fuck up raising my kids, especially because of the generational cycle. Even today I make mistakes. However, because of my self-care practice, I can look through the lens of love at my kids or my husband, to see and listen to what it is that I may be doing that is upsetting to them. Years ago I would have put up my guard and started debating and arguing, because I would have felt like I was being attacked. Now, I know that I am not in control of other people's feelings and they have a right to their own feelings, even if I don't see their point of view or agree with them. I am willing to work and give myself grace so that I can be a better mama and wife, while also holding my own boundaries. Boundaries are the key to self-care and communication is the key to boundaries.

Let's get back to what a selfish person is. A selfish person is a person who only cares about themselves. They come and go as they please. They only do what they want when they want with no regard for anyone. A selfish person has a "fuck you" attitude. You and I both know you are not selfish. If you were, you wouldn't still be reading this book. You go to the ends of the earth to make sure everyone and everything is taken care of. You give everything you've got to everyone.

If you were selfish you wouldn't worry about if the house was clean or the lunches were packed or if dinner was prepared, or the family vacation wasn't planned, or the kids went to bed happy, or your partner was sexually satisfied, or you're following the bank account budget. You wouldn't take the smallest piece of chicken that you prepared for dinner, because you want to make sure everyone's bellies are full. You wouldn't put off buying something for yourself like new underwear, because your kid wants the latest new toy. Does any of that ring a bell for you?

So, how are you enjoying those pairs of underwear that are stretched out with holes in them anyway? Like I said, a selfish person doesn't give a fuck about anyone but themselves. When you practice self-care, you mindfully take care of all of your responsibilities with love and affection along with mindfully taking care of yourself with just as much love and affection. Will people get mad at you from time to time if you say no to them, because you are doing something for yourself? Yep, but that is okay. When you practice self-care you learn to create boundaries with a kind heart. You learn that their frustration and anger is rightfully their own shit to deal with, not yours. This is because their reaction is them being triggered by something within themselves that they haven't resolved yet, or they are so comfortable in the habit that you have created with them that they are now in fear of losing that comfort.

Yes, you read that right. You do play a part in the habits that have been created and the boundaries with your family and your friends. A habit is something that you do over and over again, usually to the point where you don't even have to think about it or consciously be aware you are doing it. Everything we do is a habit from what time we get up in the morning to how and when we brush our teeth.

Our habits will change over time depending on the seasons we are in. Remember the days when you didn't have children and you could sleep in on the weekends? Then along comes the baby and you are waking up at the ass crack of dawn. Although we didn't choose the time to wake up, we chose parenthood. When I teach my clients about habits, especially in my boundary classes, I often use this scenario to explain just what I mean. Imagine you are the person in your family who always cooks dinner and dinner is always promptly served at 5:00. Then one day you learn there is a new yoga class at 5:00 on Thursdays at your favorite yoga studio, and you really want to go. Yoga is your jam. It helps you not only move your body, but when you come home you feel so aligned and centered, and most of all, happy. Now what do you think will most likely happen in this scenario? Well, if you are like most women, especially us mothers, you would scratch the whole idea of going to yoga. You'll come up with about a hundred reasons why you shouldn't go and the mom guilt will settle in. You probably won't even mention it to anyone and you'll push down the idea of rolling out your mat and tuck it away.

That's until one of those breezes starts to blow. Remember how I said our family and friends are not the cause of the tornado storm, but they could be a small breeze that begins the storm? In this scenario, you most likely will place dinner on the table and either someone will have a snarky remark about what the choice of menu for that day is or someone will sit down late to dinner and the breeze starts to blow as you begin to brew inside, muttering the words, "What about me?" And out of nowhere your mouth starts spinning like a funnel.

During this tornado storm you blurt out how you cooked this meal for them and nobody cares about you or what you want, and that you could be peacefully laying on a yoga mat right now. Nobody will know what you're talking about, because you never mentioned it. Now a selfish person would put their middle finger up and tell their family to fuck off. A person who practices self-care has self-awareness to know how important this class is to themselves and they have healthy boundaries with their family. A person who practices self-care would sit their family down and calmly explain to them that there is a yoga class that they would like to attend. Then she will take care of her responsibilities and offer to either prepare dinner for them and they can eat without her or they could eat at different times on Thursdays. Regardless, that person would go to yoga and make sure their family was fed. That person may get some push back and that's okay, because that dinner time every night is a habit that person created in their home. That person kept feeding their family every evening at 5:00, so their family expects dinner on the table at 5:00. Habits become comfortable and are difficult to give up, especially if they have been practiced for a long time. But habits can be broken and habits can change. Over time the family will have created a new habit on Thursday nights and not even realize as time goes on that their habit is now totally different. Who knows, maybe someone else in the family will make dinner on Thursdays instead. Don't chuckle, it can happen, especially if you communicate your needs and wants and stop being everyone's doormat. I see you, people pleaser!

What I like to ask my clients at this time is, "What if your child came to you and said that baseball practice or gymnastics is now at 5:00 on Thursdays? Would you even hesitate to change dinners on Thursdays?" The response is always no and my response is always, "Then, why can't you do that for you?"

I mentioned mom guilt earlier and I really want to touch base on this. Whether you are a mom or not, we always feel guilty for something around the people we love. We don't want to offend them or hurt their feelings by not complying with what they want us to do or what we think they want from us. This is an expectation brought on by them and sometimes we create the expectation ourselves.

We also think of guilt as a bad thing. Guilt, especially when we bring it on ourselves, isn't a bad thing. How could loving someone so much that you don't want them to be upset be something so wrong? However, how we allow ourselves to live our lives around this guilt can be wrong.

I know how gut wrenching it can be to leave your child, even if it is for an hour especially when they are little. Nevertheless, if I could go back in time, I would have left my kids more. I would have left them with the people I knew they were safe with and loved by and made time for myself. I loved every minute of raising my kids when they were little, but guess what? They grow up. They become adults. They leave you.

Remember what I said about when you put your head on your pillow at night all you have is yourself? Your kids grow up and they leave your home to live their own adult lives. Then you are left wondering who you are and where you go from there. When you become so consumed with being a mom, you forget to take time for yourself and you lose what your identity is to yourself. You forget who you are without them. I promise you that if you miss a soccer game, or go to the gym one morning a week or a painting class on the weekend, or make an appointment to see your therapist, your kids are going to be just fine. You should not feel guilty for doing things that not only make you feel better but make you better.

One night, after teaching my Gentle Yoga class, one of my students came up to me. She is a young mom who is a nurse with two kids under the age of three. She said, "I love coming here every Tuesday. It sets me up for my whole week. When I go home I'm not cranky and I'm relaxed, and that carries me through the rest of the week. I am nicer and have more patience with my husband and my kids."

Don't feel guilty for giving yourself moments to fill your cup up. Your family will actually appreciate that when you return home, you are more present and calm with them. Also, don't you want to teach your kids how to take care of themselves by being a role model instead of being a screaming lunatic who is overwhelmed and burnt out?

CHAPTER TWO

Why Self-Care?

Overwhelmed. Burnt out. Tired. Stressed. These are all adjectives most women, especially moms, use to describe their current state. Most moms wake up in the morning and maybe they pour themselves a cup of coffee and then they spend the majority of the rest of the day tending to everyone else. Whether you're a stay at home mom or you work in a corporate office or a nurses' station or a classroom, you are constantly revolving your life around everyone else, especially your children from their nap schedules to their preschool schedules to their primary, middle, and high school schedules. Don't forget the hours you spend in your car as an Uber service, driving your kids back and forth to sporting events and activities. Oh, and their social lives with the sleepovers and birthday parties. Add in to the mix visiting your parents and other various family members. Then there are the holidays and the birthday parties and the wedding or baby showers.

I get it, you're busy. You never have time for yourself. But I bet you have time for that glass of wine you pour every night when the kids go to bed. Or the time to scroll mindlessly through social media. Or time to go to the cabinet and grab four Oreos promising yourself you would only eat four, then twelve Oreos later, you're shaming yourself. Or the time you plopped your ass on the couch and mindlessly binged a series on Netflix, and now it's 1:00 in the morning and you need to be up by 5:00 a.m. I promise you that you do have time for yourself during the day, you are just choosing not to make it for yourself.

I believe that we have the idea of self-care all wrong. We think that we need these huge chunks out of our day for self-care. We think that self-care is going to the nail salon every two weeks or a girl's night out or going to a spa every now and then. These are all wonderful forms of self-care and are things that should be practiced within your self-care practice, but they are only once in a while. Just like anything else we do in life, if it's not consistent it will leave gaps and voids. It will feel good in the moment, but then as time goes on, without the consistency, you will start following bad habits and rituals that don't fill your cup. You'll find things to numb yourself thinking you are filling your cup like that third glass of wine or scrolling on Instagram, neither which will serve you well later. I know in the moment those things might feel like self-care, but when you practice self-care you want to look at what you are doing at the moment and ask yourself, "Will this habit or ritual help future 'me'?" For example, how will you feel after the wine wears off? My guess is that your head will feel groggy, you may have a slight headache, and your energy will be low. How is feeling that way helping you or anyone else? It's not helping anyone.

I am not here to be the wine police for moms. I enjoy my wine as much as anyone else and so should you if you choose to drink wine. However, because I have been practicing self-care for so long that I can now look at an action and question if that action is a good idea and if it will help me or hurt me. What I mean by helping or hurting is deciding if this action is going to fill my cup or empty my cup.

As I stated earlier in the book, what I have found self-care to be is practicing daily habits and rituals throughout the day that continuously fill your cup up; mind, body, and spirit. When your cup is continuously being filled it will never become empty, therefore leaving you with a fulfilled life that is healthy and happy.

There are five areas of the self that I have created habits and rituals around that I practice daily. These areas are the physical self, social self, emotional self, intellectual self, and the spiritual self. We will discuss these five areas in the next chapter. I have found that when these five areas of the self are tended to on a consistent basis, then my life flows nicely. I also have found that when something external causes chaos or grief in my life, the habits and rituals that I practice in my daily self-care practice keep me grounded, giving me strength to power through even the worst seasons of my life. My habits and rituals have also helped keep me focused and in the moment of some of the most fantastic times in my life. If it wasn't for my self-care practice, I honestly think I would have lost my mind during many seasons of my life, especially living through the pandemic and the last few years of my mom's life. I truly and wholeheartedly believe it was because of my self-care practice that I could sit next to her bedside in the hospice center and witness her take her last breath and not lose my fucking mind.

We are constantly looking at what comes next in life instead of being present in what is happening now in every aspect of our being. We want to be smarter, richer, have our stomachs flatter, our asses tighter, and our relationships more loving. We are living in a society of instant gratification, but we are never in the moment to even enjoy it. We are always three steps ahead of where we are right now. At this moment right now, I want you to practice this exercise:

- First finish reading this chapter. You may want to take notes on the directions, then put down the book, use all of your senses, and answer these questions.

- What do you see? Are you in your living room? What color are the walls? Is there sunlight coming in from the window making shadows on the walls?

- Now, what do you hear? Is there glorious silence? Is the dog barking? Do you hear your kids giggling or screaming in the other room?

- What do you smell? Did you light a candle and the

relaxing scent is filling the room? Did the dog fart and you need to cover your nose?

- Next, what do you feel? Are you still holding the book in your hands? Is the book heavy? Is the cover smooth?

- Lastly, what do you taste? Did you just have a sip of coffee or tea and the taste is still lingering on your tongue? Or maybe you have been sipping wine and you feel the warmth of that sip still in the back of your throat?

This, my friend, is called "pausing" and it is the number one tool I use every day to bring myself in the present, in the now. The practice of pausing is how I bring myself back into my body and into my consciousness. When I pause, I am becoming aware of what is in my space. I am noticing all the things in my own little world around me. The things that are influencing me from the choices I made, like the taste of the coffee in my mug that I made for myself as I sip and enjoy. And the things that influence my life that I have no control over, like the smell of the dog's fart, in which I could make a big deal over and tell the dog she's gross or I could just cover my nose and ignore it.

Do you see what I'm getting at here? When you aren't in a perpetual motion of looking forward, you have the awareness of what is happening in that moment and are capable of calmly responding to the situation.

Pausing is a tool you can use when you're in the midst of any chaotic moment to bring yourself back into your body and into the now. You can even use this tool with your kids. Teaching your kids the tools you use as an adult to self-regulate your emotions prepares them to have a toolbox already filled as they become an adult. I mean, honestly think of the world we could live in if adults were taught as children how to self-regulate their emotions, instead of sitting with a therapist for the first time in their thirties trying to undo all the shit they pushed down inside themselves as a child. Imagine a world where children learned how to set boundaries, how to take care of their mental health, and how to take care of their bodies in a healthy way, not by punishing themselves by starving or pushing themselves by working out excessively.

Practice "pausing" in the morning after the struggle of getting your kids ready for school in the morning. You know, that struggle after you have entered their room for the third time yelling, "GET UP!" or listening to your kids fight over who gets the bathroom first or the argument over eggs or pancakes for breakfast and they turn down both options, or when your child melts down in front of you because they "forgot" they had a big project due that day. Ahhh, good times. I don't miss those fucking moments! I pray for those of you still in the midst of those battles.

A great time to practice pausing is when you all pile up into the car on the way to school drop off. Before you put that car in drive and roll out of your driveway, just say the word "pause" then guide your kids to use their senses. What do you see? What do you hear? What do you smell? What do you feel? What do you taste? Doing this practice will bring them back into their bodies, and you as well. It will bring you all into the present moment. Your nervous systems will have regulated, and you will all be calmer for the start of your day.

This practice can be used multiple times throughout the day. Like I said, I use it all the time. When I was teaching who I like to refer to as "the little people" in kindergarten and first grade, I had a crazy and long commute to the school. When I would pull into my parking space in front of the school I would put my car in park, and before I did anything else I would "pause". Teaching is a stressful job. I knew that the moment I walked into the front door of that school I would have to be "on" for at least the next 8 hours, which is physically, mentally, and emotionally exhausting. So, I would take that moment to come back into my body and center myself before the mayhem would begin.

Another time I would use this practice was when my mom was either in the hospital or rehab. They were really long days. I would spend my day teaching the little people and then go straight to the hospital or rehab until visiting hours were over. After spending the day with a classroom filled with five and six year olds giving them all my energy, I would be spent; but I also knew when I walked into the hospital or rehab I needed to focus to hear what the nurses and doctors had to say. I also wanted to be present for my mom and exchange positive energy. So once again, I would pull into the parking spot at the hospital or rehab and "pause" before I would enter the building.

Not only are we constantly living in a world where we are looking at what is ahead of us, we also are living in a reactive society. How often do you say, "I will be happy when (insert whatever it is) happens?" We are never looking at what is right in front of us. We are never grateful for what we have right now. You, yourself, five years ago would probably be begging for what you have right now and the person that you have become. Yet you never realize how far you have come, because you never take a moment to look back at what you have accomplished; to take in all of the good stuff because all you have focused on is what has gone wrong instead of all that has gone right. We are never satisfied, always reaching for more, and then we just keep adding more and more on thinking maybe this one new thing will change it all. My friend, that is not how it works. What happens if you build something that doesn't have a strong foundation? It eventually falls down and it is taking everything with it.

This is why self-care is so vitally important. Self-care builds that foundation for your home. Building that foundation will create a healthy and happy lifestyle for you. Self-care can and will help prevent illnesses and diseases. It can and will prevent emotional and mental breakdowns from happening. Self-care will give you something to lean on and lean into on those dark nights of the soul, when you are curled up on the floor asking God, or whatever it is you believe in, to give you strength and courage to stand back up and move forward. Self-care will give you an awareness of who you are, an awareness of what you will and will not tolerate in your life. Self-care is an awareness of what lights you up inside. Self-care will open you up to a path to fulfill your hopes and dreams.

If you practice self-care will your life be filled with rainbows and butterflies all of the time? Hell, no! But you will have more opportunities to see rainbows and butterflies. You will be able to get through the difficult times with much more ease and grace. More importantly you will be able to "pause" even in the good moments to take in all that is happening.

My oldest daughter married her high school sweetheart in October 2021. Her wedding was supposed to be held in October of 2020. Due to the pandemic, the wedding was pushed back a year and I can look back now with a knowing in my gut and in my heart that it was all divine timing.

My mom passed away fourteen days before my daughter's original wedding date. Imagine what a shit show that would have been if the wedding would have gone as planned. It broke my heart that my mom wasn't able to be there on my daughter's wedding day, but I knew she was there in spirit watching and smiling. I could have spent my entire day dwelling on the fact that she wasn't there. I could have been angry she wasn't able to watch me wheel my grandson, the ring bearer, in a little Red Flyer wagon down the aisle during the ceremony. But I wasn't and I owe that to my self-care practice.

I was able to feel all the feelings I felt that day come up and instead of pushing them aside, I let them in. I felt the ache in my heart. I allowed my stomach to flip. And instead of wishing I could say something to my mom, I just said it out loud as if her body was next to mine, because I knew her spirit was.

The morning of the wedding I created my own ritual by walking down to the beach with a picture of my mom and my daughter in my hand. I sat with my coffee and I talked to my mom letting her know I missed her and wished she was here with us. I also let her know I was so happy she wasn't suffering and to me knowing she wasn't in pain and anguish was way more important than my pain of missing her and wishing she was there.

Before I left the beach, an orange butterfly flew by me signaling to me she was there with me and in that instant I knew that this was going to be one fucking fantastic wedding. It was! The entire day and night I would just step back and "pause" taking in all the things from the day. I used all of my senses from the taste of the Prosecco to the looks of the smiling faces of the guests, the sound of the incredible band, to the smell of the floral bouquets, and the silkiness of the fabric of my daughter's wedding gown when I hugged her. I wasn't worried about what could go wrong or what was happening next. I was just present in the moment, etching memories into my brain like the shutter of a camera. Now, when I close my eyes, in my mind I teleport myself back to that moment. Since I was so present and aware, I remember even some of the tiniest details.

My self-care practice has given me a peace and a happiness in my life I never knew could exist. I can remember my son's friend asking me what I am "on" and could he have some. I still laugh out loud every time I think about him saying that. At that time, I was starting to piece together my daily self-care practice. I started to take on this serene and calm approach to life, although if you ask my family, they would say that is bullshit. But for me it was all starting to happen internally.

Now if you ask my family, they would agree I am much more

serene and calm. I was still people pleasing, but I was also not allowing other people's shit to become my shit. I was slowly shedding all the layers of my childhood and young adult life that I had wrapped around myself for comfort and for safety, even though those layers weren't particularly really comfortable or safe. They were just what I knew at the time. I was also allowing my true authentic self shine like a bright light and I didn't give a fuck what people thought of me or of what I was doing. I was returning back to loving myself. I was returning home.

It wasn't until I put together my practicum for yoga teacher training on self-care did I realize that I had created a solid DAILY self-care practice focusing on my mind, body, and spirit. This practice was not only guiding me to live a healthy and happy lifestyle, but also was a solid foundation to pull me back up when the shit hit the fan in my life and my knees dropped to the floor.

The daily self-care practice I am going to share with you isn't something that one morning I woke up and thought, "Oh I should put together a daily self-care practice and see if it works." It organically happened over time as I was creating habits and rituals to self-care. I wasn't consciously aware of what actually was happening. However, to be truly honest, when I realized that I had created a daily self-care practice that took care of the mind, body, and spirit, I wanted to share it with the world.

Shortly after I realized what my self-care practice was, life seemed to hit me with one tornado storm after another. Maybe God was saying, "Let's test it out for good measure to be sure it really works before you share it with the world." Because holy shit, did I experience some intense storms over the last ten years, and I am one hundred percent positive that if I had not practiced the habits and rituals within my self-care practice I would have lost my ever loving mind. I would have emotionally ate my way through the last ten years. I would have burnt myself out from not sleeping and constantly being on the go. I would have had constant emotional breakdowns and meltdowns from being overwhelmed and overtired. I most likely would have been constantly sick. And I sure as hell would have not survived the pandemic with my mind intact.

My daily self-care practice has allowed me time and space to be present and enjoy my family, my friends, and my life. I am present during holidays enjoying the festivities and my family, because I know how to be in the moment. I'm not worrying about what's next, nor do I have guilt if the holiday is social media perfect. I have built boundaries around family members so that I can enjoy time with the people I truly love and want to be around. I don't make plans with my friends out of obligation or expectations, but rather out of pure joy and a wanting to be with them. I take moments throughout my day to look up at the sky and watch the clouds float by while I listen to the chirping of birds. I watch leaves glide off trees as they dance in the wind. I look into the eyes of my grandsons as I tickle them and they belly laugh. I am present. I am here. I am now. That is one of the greatest gifts my daily self-care practice has given me.

We all know self-care is important. We all know we should

be taking better care of ourselves, yet we don't. As I stated before, somewhere in your life you stopped loving yourself to make yourself a priority in your day. Somewhere something happened that caused you to feel your birthright of love belongs to everyone else, but you. Maybe you had a traumatic childhood and you learned early on that your role in life was to be the good girl and appease everyone, because you didn't want to be around conflict, because your dad or mom was always fighting. Maybe you were the shy quiet girl in school who didn't raise your hand, ever, because that one time you did, the jerk in your class laughed at you after you spoke. Instead, you found safety in silence so that you didn't feel stupid. Or maybe you had something horrific happen in your life that you never spoke to anyone about because the trauma and the pain were too much to deal with. You just shoved it down so far that you lost memory of it even happening. Regardless of the reason, it happened.

Some people refer to trauma as "big T trauma" and "little t trauma". I don't like to look at trauma that way. Trauma is trauma. It causes pain and pain is pain whether you receive a small wound or not. Sometimes a paper cut hurts worse than a gaping hole. Pain causes discomfort and when we are in pain, we usually reach for something outside of us to numb it or cope with it. Maybe you drink that bottle of wine every night, because you want to numb out from all of your responsibilities. Maybe you reach for that fourth handful of Oreos, because you eat away your emotions. Maybe you choose drugs as your form of pushing the trauma away.

We all use coping mechanisms to feel better, however the majority of us choose unhealthy mechanisms to heal ourselves. These unhealthy mechanisms are like putting a band aid over a wound. The band aid doesn't heal the wound. It just covers it up. It's the work of your body that does the healing. When you practice daily self-care, you will start pulling off the bandages, expose all the wounds, allowing them to heal in a healthy way. Heal thy self = Healthy self.

When I ask my clients what they do to practice self-care, they typically respond with an answer that revolves around one part of themselves. Usually, the answers are something like going to the gym, eating healthier, or getting pampered at a salon, which are all great habits and rituals to practice self-care; however these types of habits and rituals only help one area of self, the physical self. Sometimes I'll get the answer from clients when I ask what they do for self-care that they journal or meditate or go to therapy, which again are great habits and rituals, but their answer is one dimensional, referring to only one part of themselves. Rarely do my clients relate their relationship to their higher power, whatever that is to them, as self-care. Nor do they relate reading books or learning a new craft or hobby as self-care. And they certainly don't associate their relationships with their family and friends and co-workers as self-care.

We are complex beings with multiple layers to our being. I like to refer to them as our areas of self. In those areas there is a swirling of energy. If those areas are not engaged in a positive way, the energy will become stuck and almost stagnant causing emotional, mental, and physical pain. The way to get through the pain is to do the work, and by doing the work you create a stable place for you to live; mind, body, and spirit.

You start first with creating a sturdy floor, then you add one wall, then you add a second wall, then a third wall, and then the fourth wall. Eventually all four walls will be up, and you will be able to add the roof. Inside, you will house all the necessities you will need to live a healthy and happy lifestyle.

I like to believe that when our soul decided it wanted to venture back down to earth that it chose our body to reside in. Our soul resides inside of our flesh and blood and bones and are united. We take care of our flesh and blood and bones, yet the one thing that is giving us our essence, we seem to ignore: our soul.

How do you know you are ignoring your soul? Well, are you passionate about anything? Do you feel fulfilled in life? Do you find pleasure in the little things? Are you having any fun in your life?

I also believe that when our soul is being ignored it sends us little signals, physically. Like when you have a pounding headache because you are working too much. Your soul is childlike and it likes to have fun. Your soul will take life seriously when it needs to, but your soul wants you to be creative and laugh and love freely. Your soul is energy and if the energy is not flowing properly, your soul is going to let you know by giving you chest pains, stomach aches, back pain, or joint pain, to name a few.

Our body speaks to us when our mind can't slow down the rat race and we are too busy to listen to our soul's cues. Those cues are your intuition. You know that little voice that pops up and says, "HELLO, don't cut another piece of that chocolate cake." Or "HELLO, stop talking to that friend who drains your energy with all of her negativity every time you speak to her or are around her." Or "HELLO, you need to tell your mother in law no, you won't be there for Christmas Eve dinner again this year, because you also have a family you would like to spend time with." If we keep ignoring our soul's cues, then our body will take over, and we will start having physical symptoms. Our mind will trap our soul's energy somewhere in your body until you finally listen to it. There will be times our bodies will scream so loud that sometimes it will drop us to our knees in physical pain. We may be ignoring the cue, but our subconscious isn't. That is when we start coping with unhealthy coping mechanisms; binge eating, drugs and alcohol, abusive relationships, shopping, people pleasing, etc. These unhealthy coping mechanisms lead us down a path of unhealthy habits that eventually lead us into dis-ease in our bodies, in another word, disease.

The funny thing about disease is that we all believe that it is often passed down by generation. If our parents or grandparents suffered from a disease, then we most likely will have that same disease. Genetically it will be passed along. The truth is very few diseases are genetically passed along. Most likely the disease you are suffering from that your parents or grandparents have suffered through wasn't passed down by genetics. It was passed down by the environment that you were raised in; the habits and rituals that your parents and grandparents passed down to you. The overeating of shitty food. The over drinking or drug abuse to numb the pain. Smoking cigarettes or vaping to mask anxiety. Being a workaholic so that you don't have to deal with issues in your life.

We become just like the environment we are surrounded in growing up. As a kid we didn't know any better. It was all we knew. As adults, even if we know better, we rarely find the courage to change because even if we know what we are doing is wrong, we find comfort in the discomfort. The discomfort is normal to us and in order to get rid of the discomfort something has to change.

Change is scary. When we decide to change then the people who are part of our discomfort start to become triggered and typically try to pull us back into the discomfort. For the record, comfort doesn't always mean pleasure. Comfort is the easing of pain. When we ease our pain, we are not always participating in something that is healthy for us.

I am an emotional eater, as is my father, and he has the Santa Claus belly to prove it. My food of choice to numb my emotions is anything, and I mean anything, with sugar in it. I didn't realize the hold sugar had on me until I was in my 40s and was diagnosed with a rare blood disorder called ITP.

I had already been on a healthy path of taking care of my body at that point but I really took a deep dive into my nutrition to ensure my immune system was in tip top shape. I decided to write a food journal for a week to see what exactly I was eating and how it was affecting my body. Each day, every time I ate or drank something I would write down what it was that I ate and how I felt in the moment. An hour later I would write down how I felt at that moment. Mind you, as I said I was on a healthy path so what I was eating for my meals wasn't bad at all. I didn't keep things like Oreos in my house because I knew I would eat half the bag in one sitting. However, I saw a pattern of numbing my pain with sugar and I kind of shocked myself.

I would come home from teaching the little people all day, and especially on the days I would visit my mom in the hospital or rehab, I would head to the baking cabinet and grab handfuls of dark chocolate chips and shove them in my mouth. When I noticed this pattern, I realized I had been doing this habit of grabbing chocolate chips for quite some time. I remembered shoving dark chocolate chips in my mouth before dinner because the stress of making dinner for my family as they got older was ridiculous. Nobody was happy with the dinner menu. Somehow I convinced myself that the chocolate chips weren't really candy and they weren't in a cookie, so having a few handfuls of them wouldn't be bad, right? Around 4:00 pm, I would start shoving the chocolate chips in my mouth.

Do you see the pattern of numbing pain with something that is "comforting". I also saw this pattern on really hard days of teaching, like when I would have to escort my entire class out of my classroom, because one student was destroying my room by throwing things and ripping stuff off the wall. I would get into my vehicle while heading home at the end of the day and head straight to Dunkin Donuts to purchase a pumpkin iced coffee, because I "deserved one". Then, usually within 20 minutes, I would start beating myself up for indulging in something sugary.

Once I knew my pattern of emotional eating, I was able to begin to create new habits and rituals that were healthier to take its place. I no longer go to the cabinet and grab a handful of chocolate chips. I now have an awareness of when I am craving sugar that I am being triggered by something. Instead of shoving sugary food in my mouth to numb the trigger, I work through that trigger. I ask myself where in my body am I feeling triggered and I locate it. Then I ask myself what kind of emotion am I feeling; am I happy, sad, angry, happy, etc. Then I ask myself what is causing me to feel this way. Am I stressed about having to do something? Am I scared something happened or is going to happen? Am I sad because I miss someone or because I am feeling lonely. Once I figure out where in my body I feel the trigger, what emotion I am feeling and why, I allow myself to feel the feelings. I allow whatever sensation the trigger is causing in my body to be there. I allow whatever thoughts I am having happen. I allow whatever way my body needs to release the trigger, whether it's through tears or laughing or screaming or moving my body. Usually the sensation subsides quickly and I do believe it is because I give it permission to be what it is without me condemning or shaming it. I don't push it aside. I don't run from it. I allow it to be. The trigger no longer has control over me because I now have control over it.

When the trigger has subsided, I always feel a sense of relief and then I go on about my business. There will be times when the trigger is so immense that I do need to add extra support in processing through it. For example, I was extremely triggered the last week of my mom's life when she was in hospice. At that point, I just wanted to grab anything and everything that had sugar in it to comfort myself. I mindfully allowed some indulgances and was very aware of when I did. But when the emotions became so overwhelming I would often use a tool that has been a game changer for me.

The tool is called a heart hold. I use this tool often with my clients when I am teaching them to send love to themselves while bringing themselves into the present moment and calming their nervous system. You place one hand on your heart, whatever hand feels best for you. By placing your hand on your heart you are signaling to yourself that you are sending love. Then place the other hand on your belly, signaling to yourself that you are present. Once your hands are in place, you will take long deep inhales through your nose and release long deep exhales out of your mouth. As you continue these long deep inhales and exhales while in this hold your nervous system begins to regulate and within a few breaths you begin to feel your body and mind align and relax. At that point your trigger no longer feels like it has a hold of you. Little side note: your triggers never have control of you. You always have the power inside you to take control of your triggers, just like Dorothy in the Wizard of Oz.

I think as moms we all at some point feel like Dorothy in the Wizard of Oz. We get so wrapped up in other people's lives, especially our children, that we look for others to fill up our cups with courage and love and knowledge instead of finding it within ourselves. There is nothing that lights me up more than making someone happy, especially my kids and my husband. Not because I want the accolades of being the person who made them happy, but because I want them to live each day with a smile on their face and in their heart. I don't want them to suffer or be in pain. I want more than anything for them to be healthy and happy. That's what I believe most, if not all, moms want for their families.

However, somewhere down the yellow brick road of helping our families find their courage and their heart and their knowledge, we totally forget about ours. We don't do this on purpose. It's something that gradually happens. We begin creating habits and rituals that put everyone else before us, then eventually we are muttering those words again...*What about me? When is it my turn to work on my hopes and dreams? To chase that career? To get an education? To hang out with my besties doing the things we love? To dive into a passionate hobby that lights my soul on fire? When? When is it my turn?* And this, my friend, is when the wind starts to pick up and the breezes start to blow and along comes the tornado.

I bet if I were to ask you what are your hopes and dreams, what do you REALLY want out of life, you probably don't have a fucking clue. Much like Dorothy you are lost on a path. When was the last time you thought about something you really wanted for yourself? When was the last time you not only thought about something but spoke about it? Probably never, right? You don't have time for that. You have to pack lunches and Uber kids to soccer practice and get dinner on the table after working a full day at work. Who has time to think about themselves? You, my friend, you do. Because the packing of the lunches and Ubering the kids to soccer practice and making dinner, you create all of that by doing it all by yourself without asking for help. You do that without delegating tasks and chores around the house. You take on all the responsibilities believing you have to do it ALL. I was you, my friend. I did it all, because I thought, as a woman and mom, I was supposed to.

New mamas, I want you to listen very carefully. When your baby is placed in your arms you will do ANYTHING to keep that baby healthy and happy. That means you are going to need to ask for help. You can, but you do NOT need to do it all. There is no shame in asking someone when you can barely keep your eyes open to hold your baby so that you can take a nap. Or when you haven't showered in 48 hours, let someone hold the baby and go take a shower. Taking care of yourself is just as important as you taking care of your baby. Taking care of your life necessities is not selfish. It is necessary. Don't you want to be able to give your baby all of you, instead of pieces of you, because you're so damn tired you can barely keep your eyes open?

When you are a new mama and you start from the very beginning taking care of your well-being along with taking care of your baby's well-being, you are setting your baby to grow into an adult who will know their self worth, and know how important it is to fill their own cup up. Trust me, I know how difficult it is to be away from your child. I raised three of them. I would give anything to go back in time to when they were just little tiny humans, because I just absolutely loved that age. If I could do it all over again, I would have asked my husband to participate more in the daily routine of taking care of them. But that wasn't how I was raised. I didn't really know any different. I knew women worked, but the women I knew who worked did so out of necessity because they either didn't have a husband or their husband didn't make enough money to support their families. As I stated earlier, I was raised in the 70s and 80s. Us women of that generation watched our mothers, aunts, and grandmothers take on the majority of the responsibilities of the household, which included the cooking, the cleaning, and the caring for the children, even if the woman had a job.

Life was much different back then. Women typically had jobs but not careers. It wasn't until the 90s that I noticed the world started to shift. There were fewer and fewer stay at home moms. If you were one of them, you were considered basically a slacker. Women who worked outside of the home either looked down on you for not working or were jealous because they wished they could be home with their kids. Being a stay at home mom isn't for everyone. I know some women who were chomping at the bit to get back to work after their maternity leave was up and I know some women who almost had a nervous breakdown because they had to go back to work. If I had to do it all over again, I one hundred percent would be a stay at home mom. I don't regret that decision one bit. However, I would have done things differently.

I'd like to set the record straight though for a moment. My

husband was and still is a great father. He wasn't an absent father and made sure he was doing all the things he needed to do in his fatherly role. He is far from perfect and totally unconventional, but honestly, he pretty much nails the father role for our kids. With all that being said, when it came time for feedings, diaper changes, baths, and all those day to day mundane routines, I did the majority of it. If I asked him to do something he would do it without hesitation. But that's the thing. I had to ask. As I said earlier, while we were growing up, dads rarely did those things. Not to mention, I wasn't good at asking for anything for myself, so I just did it all. I didn't know how to set boundaries for myself. I didn't know how to use my voice.

CHAPTER THREE

Boundaries and Communication: Keys to Self-Care

Boundaries are the key to self-care and communication is the key to boundaries.

Definition: **boundary**: *noun*
  "a line that marks the limits of an area; a dividing line"[1]

Boundaries can be described as how emotionally close you let people, places, or things get to you and where you draw the

---

1   Google's English dictionary provided by Oxford Languages

line within the relationship to those people, places, or things. Boundaries say how much you are willing to give or take before asking for a change or deciding to call it quits completely. In essence, boundaries are the ultimate act of "self-love".

A boundary empowers you to take charge of your life. Nobody is in charge of your life, but you. Your yeses and your nos control the outcome of how you live your life. Boundaries free you to live life on your terms. Without boundaries, you can lose yourself, you can lack self-esteem, you can be taken advantage of, and you can burnout. Lack of boundaries can also result in emotional and mental breakdowns or even health issues.

When you don't set boundaries you will find yourself doing things out of guilt or obligation, rather than practicing self-love. Where are my people pleasers again? When you set boundaries you will find you have lower stress levels, higher self-esteem, and overall, live a healthier and happier lifestyle. I personally like to think of boundaries as my bodyguard to karma.

Karma is a chain of reactions to the things we do and say, and also a chain of reactions to the things we don't do and say. I will use the holidays as an example. For years, I would spend my holidays jamming in seeing all the people in my life and doing all the things in one day. At the end of the day, I karmically created a very exhausting day in which I did not get to enjoy my time with the people I love. I complained and complained about this for years, yet every time the holiday season came along, I would once again, out of obligation and keeping the peace with family members, jam everything into one day.

A few years ago, I finally spoke up to my husband about this. To be honest, I always felt my side of the family was being slighted, because we always were with his family for the holidays. Luckily for me, my husband understood and agreed with what I was saying and how I felt. So now we both look at a holiday as a season, not a day. We still work around other people's schedules; however, if we don't see a person on the actual holiday, we don't get upset. Now that doesn't mean that the other people might not get upset, because they do. But here's the thing. That is their shit, not yours. You are setting a boundary in a way that makes you feel happy and comfortable while still lovingly working with the other person to hopefully make them feel happy and comfortable as well. Their expectations are not your problem.

Boundaries are personal to you. This is why they are called personal boundaries. Personal boundaries are not what other people think your boundaries should be. Instead, they are limits and rules you set for yourself within relationships with people, places, things. A person with healthy boundaries when they want to can say "no" with compassion and respect towards what they are holding that boundary around and towards themself.

Here are 8 areas you may need personal boundaries around:

1. **Physical Boundary**: This is your personal space, your privacy, and your body. You may be comfortable with public displays of affection such as hugging, kissing, and hand holding. Or you may be someone who prefers to not be touched in public.

2. **Emotional or Mental Boundary**: This is your feelings.

You may not feel comfortable talking about your feelings to your friend or your partner. You may be someone who needs time to process your emotions before feeling comfortable to even share. Or maybe you are someone who needs to talk to a therapist or counselor because you need someone outside of your circle to listen to you.

3.   *Spiritual or Religious Boundary*: This is your faith. You may feel called to share your faith with everyone in your life. Or you may not feel comfortable sharing your beliefs at all and like to keep them private.

4.   *Financial and Material Boundary*: This is about your money and possessions. You may feel comfortable spending your money on family and friends and sharing your possessions. Or maybe you are a saver who likes to live a modest lifestyle and you don't want people sharing your possessions.

5.   *Time Boundary*: This is the time you give to others and to yourself. Maybe you are someone who likes to devote most of your time to being with others or to your job. Or maybe you need daily quiet time to gather your thoughts, process your emotions, and work on yourself.

6.   *Intellectual Boundary*: This is your thoughts and beliefs. This is where you like to be respected for your ideas and opinions even if they are different from others, because you like to share your thoughts and beliefs. Or maybe you are someone who likes to keep your thoughts and beliefs private.

7. *Sexual Boundary*: This is your expectation when it concerns intimacy. You may be uncomfortable with sexual comments or certain ways of being touched. Or maybe you are a free spirit with intimacy.

8. *Non-Negotiable Boundary*: This is your hard core boundary. There is no way you are crossing the line. You may be in recovery and do not want to go to the bar with your friends for happy hour. Or maybe you attend church every Sunday so you are not available for Sunday brunch with your friends.

A good example of personal boundaries would look like this. A friend asks you to dinner for Friday evening but you have had an exhausting week and all you want to do is go home, put on sweats, and binge Netflix. Immediately you feel guilty, because you don't want to hurt your friend's feelings. Here is where you set the boundary. Check in with yourself using body wisdom. Body wisdom is a tool you can use when you are having difficulty making a decision, especially around a boundary. Your body has a tendency of talking to you and revealing things before your brain reveals it. This is why you get headaches, stomach aches, and tension in the shoulders. Your body tells you something isn't right, because your brain won't stop long enough to realize something is wrong. Eventually something uncomfortable is created in the body to tell you that you need to slow down and listen. Your body won't play tricks on you like your mind will. Your mind will try to over analyze and rationalize. Let your body decide what it is you really want and, more importantly, want to do.

This is how to use body language. Place your hand on your heart. Take a few deep breaths in your nose and exhale out the mouth. Close your eyes if it is comfortable for you. Envision yourself in the decision. (ie: going somewhere, doing something, buying something, or eating something) Place yourself in your mind in that decision as if you are doing it. See yourself. Now, let your body speak. If your body leans forward or you feel an energetic pull in your chest/belly, then your body is telling you YES DO IT! If your body leans backward or you feel an energetic pull in your back, your body is telling you NO DON'T DO IT! It's not for your highest good.

If the answer is yes, then go. But if the answer is no, here is how you can set the boundary: "I would love to come, but I have had a long week and I really need some down time. But I would love to meet you Saturday night for dinner or Sunday for brunch." Here you are being honest, using your voice, and setting the boundary while being compassionate and respectful to your friend. They now know why you said no, and also know that you value their time and still want to see them when it works for BOTH of you.

You have to use your voice! People will not know your boundaries unless you tell them. Other people can not read your mind and will never know how you feel or what you are thinking unless you communicate with them. When you don't communicate your thoughts and feelings, resentment and anger can build up within yourself. You may also feel disrespected. Often the end result is an emotional breakdown filled with anger and/or sadness.

These breakdowns can be prevented if you use your voice to communicate your boundaries so that the other person or persons are aware of your thoughts and feelings. A perfect example of this is the story I shared earlier about going to a yoga class at 5:00 on Thursdays when your family is expecting their dinner on the table prepared by you at that time. Your boundaries should also be very clear. "No." is a sentence, and you do not need to apologize or explain your no when you say it. But it is important to clearly communicate your no. When you set a clear boundary you will not leave the other person wondering what it is you are thinking and feeling. The clarity of your communication will help everyone involved, including yourself. There will be no questioning where your line is drawn.

Here are some examples of clear boundaries:

1. *Time Boundary*: "I can only stay for an hour" or "If you're going to be late, please let me know ahead of time" or "I cannot attend. I already have previous plans" or "My office hours are from 9-6 Monday-Friday. I will get back to you during those hours."

2. *Intellectual Boundary*: "I don't have the answer to help you with (insert their request) right now, but maybe (insert this resource) can help."

3. *Emotional Boundary*: "I understand you're having a hard time and I want to be there for you, but this is triggering for me and I don't feel comfortable talking about it."

4. *Personal Space Boundary*: "It makes me feel uncomfortable when you (insert a touch or action). If you can't respect my space, I'll have to leave."

5. *Spiritual or Religious Boundary*: "I'm not aligned with that thought (or belief) and I would prefer to change the subject."

6. *Mental Boundary*: "I understand we see things differently and I respect your opinion, but please don't force it on me." or "I don't find those types of comments funny."

7. *Financial or Material Boundary*: "Please ask me first before borrowing my (insert possession)" or "I would appreciate it if you didn't touch my (insert material thing)" or "I don't feel comfortable loaning my money out to anyone."

8. *Social Media Boundary*: "I don't feel comfortable with you posting that on my Instagram."

9. *Non-Negotiable Boundary*: "This is a non-negotiable boundary for me and the answer will always be no."

After communicating your boundary with someone you should never feel like you need to follow up the boundary with a reason why you set that boundary. Your reasons are valid because they are your reasons. Not everyone will understand or respect your boundaries and that's okay. You need to remind yourself that their issues are not your issues. Often when people become upset or frustrated when you set a boundary it is because you are reflecting back a part of them within your boundary that is unresolved within themselves. Typically that part is unresolved trauma that they haven't dealt with and your boundary may be triggering to them. Regardless, if someone gets upset, it is essential to stand firm in your decision while kindly reminding them of your wants and needs.

Again, their emotions are their emotions, not yours. Their issues are not your issues. A good example of this would be if a family member has invited you to a family get together. However, there is a person in the family who is also invited that you are not comfortable around and need a hard boundary with. After you have politely declined to the person inviting you, they begin to either gaslight you or guilt trip you. Here is where you set the boundary by saying, "I appreciate the invitation and I am sure everyone will have fun; however, this is an event I do not feel comfortable being at." Here you are being honest, using your voice, and setting the boundary while being compassionate and respectful. Also keep in mind, when you are setting a boundary, people will only treat you the way you allow them to treat you. Boundaries are not easy, but they can be made and you don't need nor deserve to take someone's shit over them.

We often think about boundaries as only being around people and places. We can also set boundaries around things. I mentioned earlier my love of Oreos. I mean, come on, who doesn't love a double stuffed Oreo? They are fantastic! I love them so much that if I had a bag of Oreos in my home, they would be gone in two days. Hand on my heart, no lie, I would have been the one who ate them all. My husband doesn't have a sweet tooth and we are empty nesters. I can't even share them with the dogs. So, I am left to eat all the sweets that enter our home. Therefore, I very rarely buy or make sweets. Notice I said rarely. I will not and refuse to deprive myself of things I enjoy, but I know that there are times when I over indulge in the things I enjoy. So, I have created boundaries around them. Case in point, Oreos.

As I said I don't typically have Oreos in my home, but for this example let's just imagine I do have a bag of double stuffed Oreos in my house. If I begin to have a craving for the Oreos, I will check in with myself if the craving is because of an emotion or is it that I just want them. How do you know the difference? If the craving is emotionally driven you will feel like you will steamroll any family member or the dog to get to the Oreos. There is a lot of intensity in your thoughts about the Oreo and intensity felt in your body about eating the Oreo. If you are just wanting an Oreo there is no intensity in your thoughts or in your body. Intensity feels like "Fuck whatever I am doing! I NEED that Oreo, NOW!" Where no intensity feels like "I'm going to have some Oreos in a few minutes after I clean out the dishwasher."

Typically, the intense craving is caused by an emotion, because I am an emotional eater. I will locate that emotion in my body and I will work through the emotions using tools like a heart hold. I will hold my hand on my heart and belly and breathe through the emotion and the feelings that come along. If the heart hold isn't working and emotion is really intense, instead of grabbing the Oreo, I will grab a handful of blueberries or grapes to replace the craving with a healthier option. When there are those times where I just want an Oreo and it has nothing to do with emotions and everything to do with that an Oreo is delicious, I eat the Oreos. Let's be honest, it's always plural. Here I am acknowledging my wants and needs, but also have enough awareness of where I need to draw a line for myself so I am not about to do something that I know would not be in my greatest good. This, my friend, is what self-love looks like: allowing yourself the damn Oreo when you want it in a way that you know your wants and needs will be fulfilled in a healthy and happy way.

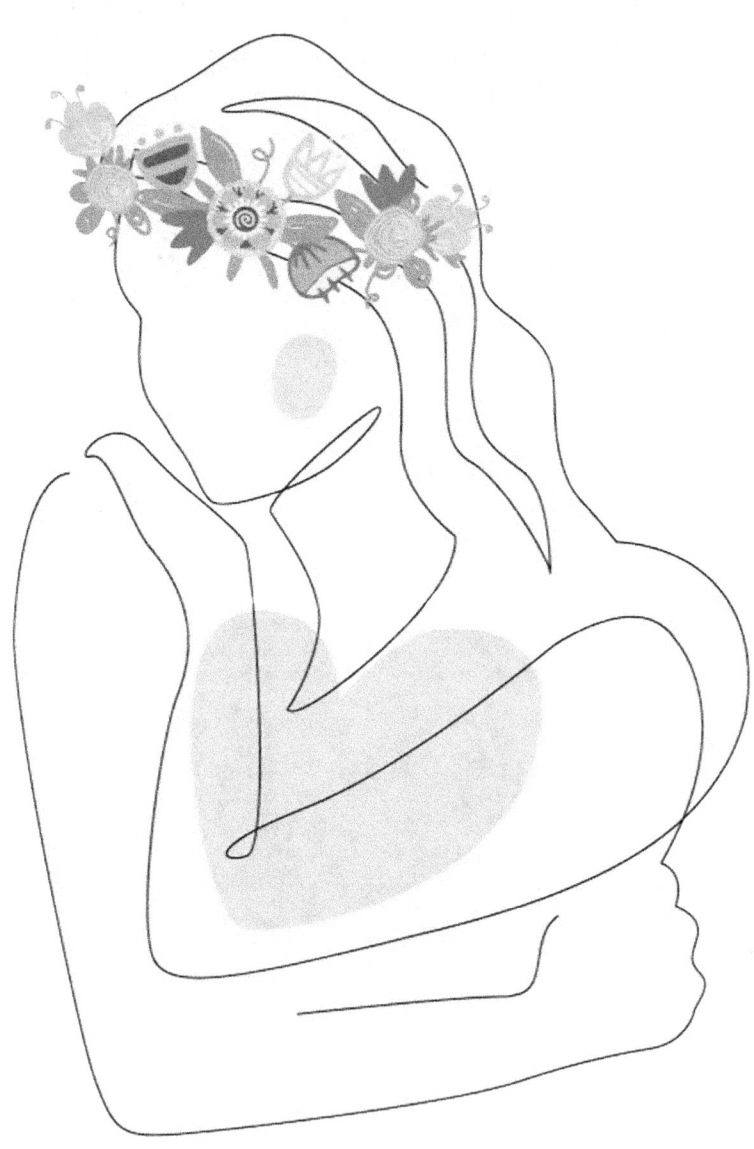

CHAPTER FOUR

The 5 Areas of Self

When someone thinks about themself, they typically think of themself as one dimensional. However, I believe people are more than one dimensional. I believe we each have areas of ourselves that make us into a whole self. Each of these areas play a vital role in who we are as a person, how we present ourselves to the outside world, and who we interact with in the outside world. Even though these areas of our "Self" are separate areas, they all need to be aligned in order to make us whole. Similar to going to a chiropractor if a section of your spine is out of alignment, it can throw your whole body and immune system off causing pain and discomfort. That is exactly what happens when one of your areas is not in alignment.

There are many areas to our Self, but in my experience, there five areas that I have found to be the most crucial. Kept in alignment, these five areas enable a healthy and happy lifestyle. They are: physical self, social self, intellectual self, emotional self, and spiritual self.

When we create daily rituals and habits around these areas of Self, we are able to live our days with much more ease, flow, and joy. These rituals and habits around these areas also are the foundation to hold us up on the difficult days.

When I ask my clients, "What do you do for self-care?" they often answer with something that has to do with their physical self, and usually it has to do with their appearance such as working out at a gym or running. Physical self does include movement, but it also includes your hydration, your sleep, and your nutrition. Taking care of your body is a lot more involved than doing crunches, and is crucial to living a healthy and happy life. Movement does not have to mean working out, although I do recommend working out at least three to five times a week, but we will discuss that later. What I mean about movement is just moving your body for at least twenty to thirty minutes a day in a way that you even slightly elevate your heart rate. Our bodies were designed to move, not sit in front of a screen all day.

I also can not stress enough how important hydration is. I tell my clients all the time that water is medicinal and water can be the answer to so many of our daily problems especially if you are dehydrated. Tired? Drink a glass of water. Hungry? Drink a glass of water. Can't poop? Drink a glass of water.

What we choose to eat can be medicinal as well. Food is supposed to be eaten for nutrition and energy to keep your body alive. Food wasn't intended to be made in a factory and packed into a box or a bag. Food can heal a body or it can destroy a body causing diseases.

The physical self also includes your sleep. I will be honest. In the physical self area the one thing I struggled with for a long time was sleep. Part of the struggle with sleep had to do with being a young mama with three babies each two years apart. But even when they got older and I could have gone to bed earlier, I didn't. I am a high energy person, even in my fifties and suffering from chronic ITP, but I was so energetic in my twenties and thirties that my twin sister nicknamed me the Energizer Bunny. For you young ones reading this, the Energizer Bunny is a character/mascot for Energizer battery commercials. Their slogan is "the battery that keeps going". My family and friends would tell me all the time to take a nap or go to bed earlier and I would respond with "sleep is for pussies." Later in therapy, I would recover why I never wanted to sleep. More on that later, too. So ideally, to take care of your physical self, you should be eating right, hydrating, moving your body, and getting rest.

When I share with people that their relationships with other people are part of their social self-care they typically respond with "I never thought about that." There are many things that the pandemic made us come to realize about life and one of them is that as humans we crave social interaction. Even if you are an introvert, it is vitally important, especially to our mental health, that we have interactions with other people daily. One of my dear friends, who is a school counselor for middle school students, was really struggling during the pandemic with her introverted students. These kids didn't have a huge social circle. They might have had one or two friends they would typically only see at school. When the pandemic hit they could not interact with them. She was seeing a massive rise in depression within these students. Shit, I was struggling as a grown ass woman not being able to see my best friends.

We need daily interaction with the people we love to keep our sanity. Yes, there are days when we all feel like we would like to be alone, and yes sometimes we all need those days. However, we need those relationships with the people who light us up inside, who walk with us hand in hand through life, keep us grounded, sometimes protected, but most of all to share our love with.

Out of all the areas, people are most confused by the intellectual self. Have you ever heard the phrase, "If you don't use it, you lose it?" Well, this is true about our brains. Our brains are designed to think and to process things. Our brains are muscles, and when we don't challenge our brains or fill them with new information, they turn to mush similar to our abs when you stop doing crunches. This is why intellectual self-care is so important.

When we were younger we were learning new things everyday and we were stimulated. As adults, life feels like the same shit just a different day. Add into the brain numbing of social media and Netflix and our brains really turn to mush. Hell, we don't even need to memorize our phone numbers anymore. Life has become so much easier with technology and modern ways, yet it's all making life harder for us, because it's turning our brains to mush.

When I ask my clients what it is they do to self-care, the second typical answer I get from them is usually "I talk to a therapist". Which is freaking fantastic! Talking to a therapist would be categorized under the emotional self. I am a huge advocate for therapy! I believe there isn't a single person walking this earth who hasn't had some kind of trauma in their life. Even if we live a pretty healthy and happy lifestyle somewhere, somehow, something negative happens in our lives.

We can't control the outside forces of things that happen to us, but we can control the way we respond to them. Typically, during and after a traumatic experience, we shove that trauma right down into our bodies and just let it sit there, festering. Therapy guides us through our trauma so that we can learn to live with the trauma instead of avoiding it and numbing it out with bad habits and rituals causing us to live an unhealthy and unhappy lifestyle. Therapy also allows us to just talk to someone who isn't invested in our lives, so they can remove emotion from the conversation.

There are many different types of therapy and my favorite type of therapy is talk therapy. When we talk to our friends and family they want to help us and what I mean by helping us is to fix us or fix the situation. When in reality we just want someone to listen to us. Therapists will listen without judgment and will allow us to figure out the process on our own. Plus, they give us tools to help along the way.

When I refer to spiritual self, I am not referring to religion, unless your spiritual self follows a religion, then by all means follow that path. However, there are many people, including myself, who do not identify with one religion. When I was born, my parents baptized me as Presbyterian. We only went to church for weddings, funerals, and baptisms. My mother was forced to go to church as a child and as an adult she refused to go. Even though my dad was and still is of Christian faith, he always had a spiritual connection to his God that had nothing to do with the bible. My dad's spiritual connection grew stronger while he was in the Vietnam War witnessing some of his army buddies lose their lives. Even as a young child, I had that same spiritual connection as my dad. He would teach Christianity to myself and my sister with the majority of his teachings about Jesus, typically around the holidays. All in all, to me Jesus just seemed as if he was a cool dude who just wanted to spread love, break bread, and drink wine. I can totally relate to wanting to spread love and I do love me some bread and wine.

As a young child I just had a knowing there was something more out there. I would have conversations with God all the time. I went to bed and would say my prayers in my head. "Now I lay me down to sleep I pray to the Lord soul to keep. If I should die before I wake I pray to the Lord my soul to take." Then I would bless my family and friends. As I became older my connection grew stronger and stronger.

That spiritual connection got me up off the ground from the fetal positions more times than I can count. Like the time I was told I would never be able to have children. Then surprisingly finding out four months later I was pregnant which happened to be six months before my wedding that I had been planning for four years was supposed to take place. Or the time when both my daughters were born premature and were in the NICU, and I was discharged from the hospital and had to leave without my babies. Or the time when my husband had a heart attack as we were standing in MoMA in NYC looking at the art on the wall. Not to mention the time when I was diagnosed with a rare blood disorder called ITP and had to wait a week for all the test results to come back to rule out cancer and leukemia.

A spiritual self-care practice gets you through the really fucking hard times. But a spiritual self-care practice also makes you extremely grateful for the big and little things in life. Like watching your children interact with their own children to noticing a leaf glide down off a branch dancing in the wind.

In the next few chapters I will go into more detail about each of these areas of self and why it is important to have daily self-care habits and rituals around these areas. I will also give tips and tools on how to incorporate these habits and rituals in each of these areas. As a side note I want you to understand that these habits and rituals are the habits and rituals that work for me. Your habits and rituals within the five areas do not have to be the same as mine; however, I encourage you to give them a whirl if you feel called to. If the habits and rituals aren't for you then by all means don't use them and please do not compare my self-care practice to yours. We are all unique individuals, and therefore our self-care practices should be uniquely our own.

With all of that being said, I truly believe that to be aligned mind, body, and spirit, we must focus each day on all five areas of self: physical, social, emotional, intellectual, and spiritual. I know it seems like a lot and you're probably rolling your eyes at me thinking, "Who is this chick telling me to self-care on five areas of myself when I barely have five seconds a day to piss by myself?" But I promise you, having a daily self-care practice focusing on all five areas is not as difficult as it may seem. Plus, many habits and rituals overlap into different areas. Sometimes you can knock two things out with one habit or ritual!

In case you are wondering what's the difference between a habit and a ritual, let me clear that up for you. A habit is something you do repeatedly for the purpose of performing the action itself, like brushing your teeth. You start doing something once and then over time that action becomes so ingrained you do it with no thought about it. A ritual is something you do with deliberate intention and purpose outside the action itself, like clearing your meditation space with palo santo before you meditate. Habits are the practical side to your self-care routine whereas rituals bring in the magical side to your self-care routine. Again, this is your self-care practice so if one word does not resonate with you, then by all means don't use it.

Taking care of your whole-self, mind, body, and spirit, will bring your life to a whole new level. You will have such an increased amount of self-knowledge, because when you practice your daily habits and rituals you will create a self-study. Through your self-study you will begin an exploration of yourself where you will learn what brings you joy in life and what does not. This exploration will guide you into the knowing of what people, places, and things are serving you in your life and what people, places, and things you may need to let go of. You will become compassionate with yourself and you will find it easier to become compassionate with others. You will find your relationships with other people grow into a much deeper and loving way. You will see life through the lens of love.

I work with a client who had a very loving relationship with a close family member; however, that relationship would become strained from time to time. In years past they would scream and yell at one another during arguments, then they would go months sometimes without talking to one another. Once I started working with my client and guiding her to create her own self-care practice, she began to have a self-awareness of what triggered her, but also could see triggers in other people. She began to realize that whenever she would argue and fight with the family member, it was usually because the other family member would become triggered, and it had nothing to do with my client. Their arguments would range from topics from raising their children to worldviews, but my client noticed when their family member was arguing with her, it had nothing to do with her and everything to do with her family member living in fear. Fear of being wrong. Fear of being judged. So even when a vague topic would be discussed and the family member's fear would begin to rise, she would become defensive and immediately start an argument. Having a self-care practice, my client now knew her boundaries and one of them was to not get into petty arguments. So either she would say, "We can agree to disagree and let's change the subject," or my client would just let her family member say what she needed to say and then move on to another subject. When we don't acknowledge the battle, we take away their power. It's kind of like the saying, "Don't add fuel to the fire".

One particular day there was an incident where my client realized she was going to need to amp up her boundaries with the family member. They were both at a family function and once again a discussion quickly turned into an argument. This time the family member was screaming in my client's face, poking my client in the forehead, and saying some very nasty comments to her. My client sat there quietly and allowed her family member to just purge out of her whatever she needed purged. She obviously had some pent up resentment towards my client. Eventually, other family members stepped in and removed the family member from my client's presence and they took her home. When everything calmed down, another family member asked my client why she just sat there and took that, the screaming and the poking. My client explained she could have retaliated. She could have yelled back at her and she could have even easily put her hands on her too, but in the end what would that solve? My client had learned through her self-care practice that if someone attacks you and you have done nothing except maybe disagree with them, then that attack is fear based. My client also had learned to look at people's reactions through the lens of love and curiosity and not through anger and judgment.

When we step outside of our own thoughts and emotions and place ourselves in others thoughts and emotions, we can have an understanding of the pain and suffering the other person may be in.

Clearly my client's family member had been harboring some sort of fear. When fear arises, we usually take one of three ways to approach the fear: fight, flight, or freeze. My client's family member chose to fight. Since my client had been doing the work of self-care she sat there quietly during the incident breathing long inhales and exhales out of her nose, repeating to herself, "This is fear based and this is her shit, not my shit."

Was my client pissed? ABSOLUTELY! Did my client want to haul off and punch her family member in the face? ABSOLUTELY! Did my client feel bad for her family member? ABSOLUTELY! Because once her family member's tornado storm settled, she had a lot of damage to clean up with my client and the other family members. My client just had to open up her windows and doors and let the fresh air in. She also knew that her relationship with that family member would now change, because she created new boundaries so that she would no longer be in the eye of her family member's storm again.

Learning when and how to make yourself a priority is self-care, and is one the greatest forms of self-love. It takes time to learn how to set boundaries. It takes time to learn how to say no. And it takes time to learn how to put yourself first. But when you do learn these things, you will begin to live a life of happiness beyond anything you could have imagined.

In the next few chapters I will break down the five areas of

Self, explaining in more detail why it is important to nourish and take care of these areas daily. I will also give you tangible ideas for habits and rituals for you to use in your daily self-care practice. Remember though, your daily self-care practice belongs to you, so if something does not align with you, you can change them or give them a little twist to suit you.

CHAPTER FIVE

The Physical Self

The physical self is your body and your physical self-care is how you maintain, nourish, and take care of your body. As I mentioned earlier, the physical self is broken down into four different categories: movement, hydration, sleep, and nutrition. I will be sharing with you all the tips and tools that I use for my physical self-care. Don't worry. I am not going to try to sell you a specific exercise program or tell you to follow certain fitness instructors. Nor will I tell you what fad diet to follow.

I think everyone's physical journey, when it comes to their fitness and nutrition, is uniquely different, because we are each uniquely different. For example, when it comes to fitness, depending on your body type, you will be able to accomplish something someone else may not. Someone tall with a long torso and short arms may never be able to touch the floor in a forward fold, while someone who is what I like to refer to as vertically challenged, because I am that someone, with a short torso and longer arms, may be able to lay their hands flat on the ground in a forward fold.

I would like to make a side note here about comparison. Will you please stop worrying about what everyone else is capable of and what everyone else is doing?! Comparing your journey to someone else's journey is just as mind numbing as scrolling on social media. It is a complete waste of time unless you are using that time to find encouragement and useful information to better yourself. Seeing someone else accomplish something and wanting that for yourself is amazing. Beating yourself up over not being able to accomplish something is just fucking stupid. Just because something is right for someone else does not mean it is right for you.

We have become a society that is so consumed about being like anybody else. We don't even pay attention or know who the fuck we are, what we want, or what it is we have to offer the world. You were born with your own unique, beautiful, quirky, weird, and wonderful qualities. You were put on this earth with intention and following someone else's dream is not going to allow you to fulfill your time here on earth as who you truly are meant to be. This journey of self-care will help you stop comparing yourself to other people. It will help you realize your true potential of who you are. It will help you realize the information other people are sharing with you, including myself, are lessons we have learned over the years from our guides, mentors, and teachers. We don't share because we think we have all the answers, but because we found something that worked or is still working for us. What I have learned from my guides, mentors, and teachers is a collaboration of all of their teachers, guides, and mentors, and the information they have passed along. So stop beating yourself up, because someone else is living their life one way and you tried it and it's not working out for you. Instead, change your mindset to "that just wasn't for me" and move on to something else. What I am sharing with you in this book is what has worked for me. I would love for you to try all the tips and tools I am going to share with you, but if it doesn't work, like I said before, either don't do it or find a way to tweak it so that it works for you.

MOVEMENT:

Okay back to the physical-self. When I refer to movement I am not referring to "workouts" even though I do believe every person should have some sort of workout routine. When I refer to movement, I am referring to getting your ass up off the chair or the couch and not being sedentary. On an average day, a person should be walking at minimum 10,000 steps a day and should move their body for 20-30 minutes a day where they slightly elevate their heart rate. Our bodies are meant to move and I wholeheartedly believe in the saying "a body in motion stays in motion". When we do not move our bodies, then our bodies begin to lose muscle. We lose stamina. We lose strength, but also we begin to lose our brain power. Everything within us is interconnected. When we move our bodies by moving our arms and legs in a bilateral motion even just by walking, we are sending frequencies to our brain to transfer thoughts from one side of the brain to the other and then our thoughts become ping pong balls back and forth.

This is why runners refer to running as therapy. During their run, the movement of their arms swinging back and forth along with their legs alternating as they step sends the frequency of thoughts back and forth, allowing the person to process their thoughts, feelings, and emotions. When we feel "stuck" what is actually happening is the thoughts and emotions become trapped on one side of the brain. The thoughts and emotions won't move, but when we move our body, we give those thoughts and emotions a gentle nudge, and they begin to become unstuck.

We also begin to feel happy when we move our bodies. When we move our bodies, we release endorphins which are referred to as happy hormones. Endorphins can help relieve pain in your body and mind, they can reduce your stress level, and basically just improve your sense of well-being. Movement not only helps you physically. It also helps you emotionally and mentally.

I am not going to tell you what type of movement you need to be doing because this is your journey, not mine. Also, I am not going to tell you that you should be doing 30-60 minute hardcore workouts or become a runner if that's not your jam. If you hate running, DON'T RUN! Why would you choose to do something you hate? Choosing a movement you hate will only set you up for not moving, because within a few weeks, hell, maybe even a few days, you will just give up on it. All that matters is that you find a movement you enjoy. That is the key here!

I am going to share what type of movements I enjoy and why. Again, you DO NOT need to move your body in the way that I do. I do however encourage you to try all the things I suggest and see what works best for you. A friend of mine asked me years ago if I thought a certain exercise that was trending at the time actually worked. My response was I think all of them work, if you do them consistently and with joy.

What happens often when people start a fitness journey is they give up within two weeks and for various reasons. Maybe they are impatient and don't see the results fast enough so they just say fuck it and give up. Or their bodies are so sore from moving in a way they haven't in years, or ever. Instead of working through the discomfort they give up. Or maybe they just dread the thing they are doing. I call these people two-weekers.

It takes about two weeks for you to start feeling a difference in your body. It takes about four weeks for you to start noticing a difference in your body, and it takes about eight weeks for other people to start noticing a difference in your body. It will take months for you to see a huge difference in your body, but that's the problem. People don't want to do the work or to wait. They want a quick fix like a diet pill or supplements or a fad diet. Again, those things will work in the moment, but they are not sustainable nor are they really healthy for you. Moving your body is healthy for you!

If you started a fitness program and you gave up because you aren't seeing results, try again. If you aren't seeing results, try harder. If you are sore, take it a little easier for a day or two and jump back in it. Rome wasn't built in a day and neither will your muscles. If you dread your fitness program, change it! The key is to find something you enjoy doing.

Look, none of us actually wake up thinking, "Fuck, yeah! It's workout time." Well maybe some of you do, and kudos to you. However, most people dread starting their workout for the day, but honestly, I don't know a single person who dreads their workout afterwards. Instead, most people I know, including myself, feel really good about themselves after their workout. What I like to do to motivate myself to workout is imagine how I will feel at the end of my workouts. I cultivate that feeling in my mind and my heart, which gives me motivation. I want to feel that feel good feeling of a post workout. I also give myself the incentive of drinking my coffee after my workout. I know that cup of deliciousness is waiting for me in the kitchen, and I can smell it during my workout, which makes me move my ass faster so that I can enjoy it.

One of my absolute most favorite ways to move my body, and one of the most accessible ways that most people can incorporate movement in their day, is by walking. Yep, just by lacing up my sneakers and heading out the front door to take a walk around my neighborhood or going to a local trail at a park to get my steps in not only makes me feel better physically, but it helps me feel better mentally. When we take walks, we have that bilateral movement going on. We increase our heart rate and get all those juices flowing and pumping in our bodies.

Sometimes I put my earbuds in and listen to a podcast or music, but most times I just walk looking and listening to nature. For me nature is my "church" (more about that when we discuss the spiritual self). Sometimes I like to walk alone, but most times I walk with my husband, and we bring along our dogs, Sedona and Maddie, with us.

Fitting in 20-30 minutes of walking is easier than you think it may be. Here is the secret sauce: you don't have to walk all 20-30 minutes at once. Maybe you take a 10 minute walk in the morning and then another 10 minute walk after dinner. Maybe you take a 15 minute walk at lunch and then after dinner you take another 15 minute walk. Maybe your walk is your solitude alone time or maybe you call your bestie and meet her for a walk around her neighborhood. All of these suggestions I've shared with you are how I incorporate walking into my physical self-care practice.

Do I walk every day? No. I live in the northern east coast and depending on the season we are in, there are days it's either pouring down rain or so hot your eyeballs sweat or so god awful bone chilling cold that you won't catch me outside if my life depended on it. But you can bet your ass when the weather is beautiful or at least decent, you can find me outside watching the clouds glide by while listening to the birds sing and feeling the wind blow through my hair as I walk.

If you are wondering what my second favorite way to move my body is, I am happy to tell you. That would be the practice of yoga. Depending on the mood I am in that day or the way my body is feeling, I either like the pace of a vinyasa flow or a slower moving hatha practice. Moving my body through asana speaks to my soul. Moving through a vinyasa flow sequence or the longer hold of poses through hatha sequences brings my heart rate up, challenges my mind, while building strength but also giving my body a nice soothing stretch.

When I began practicing yoga in a studio, something inside of me just clicked. It was as if who I am as a person began to surface instead of hiding behind closed doors and windows. Sitting in a guided meditation before my practice, even if it was just for a few minutes, allowed me to quiet my thoughts long enough to realize the negative thoughts and stories I had been telling myself. After recognizing them, I was able to reframe my thinking.

Through my asana practice, I was gradually beginning to see changes within my body. I was reaching goals that I never thought were possible, like finding my way into poses like crow pose.

Yoga not only challenged and changed my body in positive ways. It also challenged and changed my mind in positive ways. Through my yoga practice, I was able to learn to accept things as they are in the moment without judgment, whether that meant physically, emotionally, or mentally. I also learned grace and forgiveness in that what we were capable of yesterday, we may not be capable of today, and that is okay. Our journey on our mat is the same as our journey in life. We are humans trying to live in this world not just one day at a time, but one moment at a time. Even when we put our best foot forward with all good intentions, things may not work out the way we had hoped. Instead of holding onto expectations of how we think something should be, when we practice yoga on or off our mat, we accept it for what it is. We allow it to be and we make the best of what it is. If we were to add friction or tension to what it is, then it will only cause harm.

For example, physically if you were to try to push yourself into a pose that your body just isn't feeling in that moment, you could cause damage to your muscle or tendons. Similarly, if you try to push yourself into an emotion, it could cause you to feel overwhelmed, frustrated, or even defeated. Yoga has taught me to meet myself where I am whether that's in my physical body or mentally and emotionally with grace and forgiveness. I also learned through savasana that it is important to allow myself to pause during the day allowing all the positive things too.

I have practiced yoga for years, but running used to be my jam. I used to run all the time, especially outside. I would feel incredible after a run. My head would feel so clear and although my legs would feel like rubber afterwards, I felt unstoppable. Unfortunately, when I was being diagnosed with chronic ITP, I refrained from running for fear of falling and hurting myself, because there was a possibility of bleeding internally if I were to hit my head or a major organ. This is a prime example of how my practice of yoga has helped me. Today I am cleared to run as long as my CBC counts are in a "safe range". To be honest though, I have tried running again like I used to, but the trauma of being diagnosed with a rare blood disease that has no rhyme or reason to when the disease will decide it would like to wreak havoc on my body again is still fresh in my mind, even though I have been dealing with this disease for almost a decade. Maybe one day I will lace up my sneakers again and hit the pavement consistently, but for now I choose to honor where I am in this journey of fitness. I honor my body where it is and I try not to compare my body to where it was a decade ago. I am not the same person I was then, so obviously my body will not be the same either.

Who you are today is not who you were five days ago, five months ago, or five years ago. This is another great lesson in comparison. You will never be that person again. So, when you stand in front of your mirror judging your body for what it is, try honoring your body instead. As long as you are not dealing with a disease or injury that prevents you from changing the way your body is, you HAVE the power to change that.

Here is the thing, my friend. Your body is not going to change until you change your mindset and get off your ass and start doing something about it. Scrolling through social media looking at fitness people or pinning workouts on Pinterest are not going to get you to your fitness goal. I also want to be totally transparent here. The goal here is not to weigh a certain weight or to fit into a certain size pair of jeans. The goal is for you to be healthy. The goal is to prevent you from things like insomnia, high blood pressure, high cholesterol, and type 2 diabetes, because all of those things for the majority of us are preventable.

It's the bad habits and rituals you choose every day that can lead you down the path of illness. I have witnessed that path with my mom and trust me you don't want to go down that path. If you have children, you sure as fuck don't want your children to watch you down that path. I don't want my kids to have to wipe my ass after I just passed out on a portable toilet that is next to my bed, because I couldn't stand up, let alone walk to the bathroom. I don't want my kids to have to drive and pick me up from dialysis, because I am no longer capable of driving my car. I don't want my kids to have to chase the ambulance to the ER and then spend days or even weeks sitting in a hospital room next to me. I don't want those things for myself or for my kids, and I am pretty sure you don't want them for yourself or your kids either.

Moving your body every day is not a punishment. It is actually a gift. Some people are not capable of moving their bodies and they would give anything to be able to. When you can't move your body, you find a whole new appreciation for what your body is capable of. When I was diagnosed with chronic ITP, I went from working out twice a day (yes, I said twice a day) and barely ever sitting down to being told to sit on the couch and not to move. I couldn't even vacuum my house or carry the laundry. I couldn't go grocery shopping or cook meals for my family. During my diagnosis of chronic ITP and the months that followed, I thought I was going to lose my fucking mind. Movement to me is medicinal. When I move my body, I not only am making myself physically stronger, but I also process my thoughts and emotions, making myself emotionally stronger.

Whether moving my body through a workout or moving my body through cleaning my house, when my body is in motion my brain begins to take all of my thoughts and place them in a single file. The best way to describe it is as if my thoughts are all gathered together facing multiple trails in the woods trying to figure out which trail to go down. Once I start moving my body, a thought will find its way to a trail and begin its journey. Then the other thoughts will either begin to follow along becoming clearer as they continue down the path, or they disappear. Eventually, these thoughts begin to make a pattern and become clearer. This is moving meditation. This is when a-ha moments happen or thoughts we have shoved down resurface to hopefully be processed.

When you learn to find gratitude for your body and begin to love your body for what it is capable of, instead of your expectations of what it should look like, you begin to appreciate your body more. You begin to treat it lovingly, not judgmentally.

One thing I do when I find myself judging my body is a ritual called "Body Love". After I take my shower and I am putting lotion on, I tell my body thank you for the things it is capable of doing for me. For example, when I put lotion on my legs I talk to my legs and give them gratitude for what they have done and still do for me. "Thank you for holding me up every day." or "Thank you for being strong so that I can hold my grandsons and carry them around."

I have always hated my legs. My legs are short and I have what I consider thick thighs. My mom would refer to them as "athletic legs" and would tell me she was always jealous of my legs, because her legs were very thin. Me, not so much. I wanted long slender legs, you know with the gap between the thighs. As I became an adult and had multiple kids, I started to get varicose veins. I had multiple surgeries to remove them, partly because of vanity, but the main reason I had them removed was they were extremely painful and itchy. Once the most painful veins were removed, I stopped with the surgeries, but many of my veins are still there along with some new ones. I used to be extremely self conscious of them, and from time to time I still am. I am human after all. Once I started practicing the ritual of "Body Love" and thanking my body for the things it can do and what my body does for me, I became less self conscious about them and started to see and feel about my legs differently. This is the body that I chose to be in on this earth and I will love it for what it is capable of and not hate it for what it is not, and certainly not hate it for what it looks like compared to other people.

Embrace who you are, not who other people are. Find your best and favorite features of yourself and focus on them instead of focusing on what you don't like. When your energy is channeled into the positive, you will only look at the positive and the negative will disappear. This ritual truly was a game changer for me in finding a way to love myself as who I am, not who I think I should be.

After I was diagnosed with chronic ITP, it took almost a year for my hematologist to be able to give me the green flag to return back to working out. Truthfully, it took me a few years to feel comfortable enough to really start working out again.

During that time, I still practiced vinyasa yoga and walked and hiked a lot. Today, I am back to a workout routine five times a week. I truly believe, especially as we age, we should be working out at least 3-5 times a week. During those workouts we should use some sort of resistance or weight training included for a minimum of 20-30 minutes a day.

I know, don't roll your eyes at me. I know I said movement isn't about workouts and it truly isn't. Movement truly is about not allowing yourself to be sedentary all day, especially if your job requires you to sit down most of the day. Just take it from someone who is in the over 50s club, you lose muscle, agility, and stamina really fucking fast as you age if you don't workout at all. Adding in a low to moderate workout a few times a week, whatever style workout you choose, that has some resistance or weight training will increase your physical health tremendously as you age. For example, if you love to walk, hold weights in your hands as you walk or put weights around your ankles. Adding the weight will add resistance, which will build your muscle.

When your body is healthy from movement, it can heal faster, and your immune system will be stronger. You will not only feel better physically, but also you will feel better mentally and emotionally, because all of those feel good happy hormones and chemicals will be flowing in your body. I'm also going to say this, which I know isn't a popular statement these days, but looks matter. Meaning, when you look good in whatever way you feel is your optimal best then things in your life begin to flow. You have more confidence; you're happier. Don't believe me? Okay, you tell me how many selfies you have of yourself in your messy bun and sweats compared to when your hair is done and you have a cute outfit on. You know I am right.

To sum up movement for the physical self:

- Move your body with a movement you enjoy in a way that slightly increases your heart rate for at least 20-30 minutes a day. This could be achieved through movement such as walking, riding a bike, or dancing. The whole 20-30 minutes of movement does not need to be achieved all at once. You could break your movement up to 10-15 minutes in the morning and then 10-15 minutes in the evening.

- You also should be taking a minimum of 10,000 steps a day. There are multiple devices you can use to count your steps for the day including your phone. Ways to get steps in are to use the stairs instead of the elevator, park your car further away in the parking lot from the building, take a lunch break walk or a stroll around the neighborhood after dinner.

- Lastly, it is not required, but it is highly recommended that for 3-5 days a week you do a low to moderate intensity workout that includes resistance or weight training to build those muscles and help with agility. As we age we become more and more sedentary which means we will have less and less muscles to protect our bones and lose our stamina quicker.

HYDRATION:

We all know when we move our body it is very important to keep our bodies hydrated especially if we are sweating during our movement. But even if we don't move our bodies, we need water and lots of it! Did you know about 70% of people are walking around dehydrated and they don't even realize it?

More than half of our body consists of water. When our body is depleted of water it affects our organs, including the brain. Hello brain fog! The obvious thing we notice when we are dehydrated is that we have a dry mouth and we feel thirsty. However, if we are dehydrated, we develop other symptoms like headaches, muscle cramps, rapid heartbeat, exhaustion, constipation, and hunger pains. What's the first thing we have been conditioned to do when we have a "symptom"? We grab over the counter products like Tylenol and Pepto Bismol when all we probably need is a glass or two of water.

Here are ways we benefit from drinking our water:

- Flush out toxins

- Support a healthy weight

- Increase energy

- Healthier looking skin

- Better digestion

- Prevent headaches

- Boost your immune system

You are probably wondering how much water you need to drink in a day. That's a great question. You could go by the good old-fashioned method of drinking 8 glasses of water a day. However, that is a generalized method assuming everyone is the same height and weight. Because we are all uniquely different, some of us may need more than 8 glasses of water. The method I like to use when gauging how much water I need to drink in a day is by drinking half my weight in ounces of water. For example, if you weigh 100 lbs, you would drink 50oz of water a day. Now if you are a caffeine coffee drinker like I am, you need to replace however many ounces of coffee you drink with that many ounces of water. The same goes for alcohol too.

You are probably now thinking if you drink that much water you are going to need to go to the bathroom a lot. Yes you are, especially in the beginning when your body is flushing out all the nasty toxins. Your bright yellow pee is one of the best gauges to tell you that you are dehydrated. Your pee should be clear. If your pee is not clear you definitely need to drink up!

I get some of you may have jobs where there are long periods of time where you can't get to the bathroom. Hello teachers, I see you! Did I mention I used to be an elementary school teacher? There is nothing worse than standing in front of a room full of students doing the pee pee dance waiting to be able to walk your students to lunch or special so that you can finally pee. Oh yeah, and the multiple trips to the gynecologist because you have yet another urinary tract infection because you had to hold your pee so long or you didn't drink enough water because you were afraid you would pee your pants during a lesson. Or in my case, you just completely forgot to drink water because you're so focused on the little people in front of you. I know the "suits of education" could care less about teacher's bathroom breaks, but when you are lucky enough to work with a fantastic staff, you can find ways for someone to cover your class while your students are working independently so that you can pee. Teacher friends don't be afraid to work with your grade level team or support staff and ask for coverage so that you can let your pee flow!

When I was teaching I would come home completely dehydrated, because I would literally just forget to drink. I would come home dehydrated even though I had bottles of water in my lunch bag.

I am going to share the hacks I learned on how to keep hydrated throughout the day while I was teaching.

- When you wake up, drink an entire glass of room temperature water or a cup of warm water with lemon. Why room temperature? If we put cold water in our bellies first thing in the morning, we are then firing up our digestive system and we don't want to do that after our bellies haven't had anything in them for hours. We want to slowly say good morning to our bellies. Another reason you would want to drink room temperature water or a cup of warm water with lemon is because if you are a coffee drinker, you are going to want to flush out your system before you add all the acid from the coffee in your belly. If I don't drink my water before my coffee, my belly likes to talk to me in the morning and it's not a pleasant conversation.

- During the day I add lemon to my water because lemon has so many benefits: lemon is a good source of Vitamin C, lemon improves your skin quality, and lemon aids in digestion. I also like to add different fruits into my water to give it some flavor. When my water tastes good, I am inclined to drink more of it.

- Here is the secret sauce to ensure you are drinking enough water: timed water bottles. When I purchased a water bottle that had the ounces and the times written on the bottle to tell me I needed to drink my water, it was a game changer! For one, I knew I drank enough water for the day if the water bottle was empty. Secondly, I was no longer just sipping my water and barely drinking the bottles of water I would bring with me to school. I was chugging that shit, because I knew by each hour how much water I needed to drink. By 2:00 pm I needed that bottle emptied so that I could fill it up for round two. If you are a visual learner like me, you need to see things in front of you. I am now a retired teacher but I still use those timed water bottles constantly, and I buy them as gifts for people. You can purchase a timed water bottle online on Amazon or in stores like Five Below. If you have family or friends who are elderly they make a great gift. I can not tell you how many times I was in the hospital with my mother and elderly people were coming in with complications to their illnesses because they were simply dehydrated. I am going to say it again, water is medicinal.

To sum up hydration for physical self-care you need to drink your water every day. Here are suggestions on how to ensure you drink your water:

- Every day drink at least half your body weight in ounces of water.

- If you drink anything that contains caffeine or alcohol you should replace those ounces with water because caffeine and alcohol cause dehydration. For example, if you drink an 8 ounce cup of coffee you should follow that cup of coffee with an 8 ounce glass of water.

- Purchase a timed water bottle to ensure you are drinking enough water during the day because it is easy to forget to drink your water when you are busy during the day.

- Chug your water, don't sip.

- Before you reach for the Tylenol for a headache or Pepto for an upset belly, drink a glass of room temperature water because more than likely you are just dehydrated.

NUTRITION:

Since we are talking about what we take into our bodies, this would be a good time to segue into nutrition. Before I type another word, I want to be sure to mention I am not a nutritionist nor am I certified in any way when it comes to nutrition. The information I am sharing with you is from years of research on how to combat a shitty immune system that I had since I was in my late teens and especially after I was diagnosed with chronic ITP in my mid forties. I have spent countless hours working with my general practitioner, my hematologist, and my nutritionist to create a healthy way of eating that is beneficial to me.

My main focus when it comes to nutrition is to keep my immune system as solid as possible so that I stay healthy. When my immune system is down, so are my platelets. My other focus when it comes to nutrition is to try to eat in a way that is preventative for diseases. My mother could have prevented her type 2 diabetes from turning her body into a war zone of other diseases. For most people, type 2 diabetes is reversible. All you need to do is change your habits of eating and move your body every day. It really is that simple, yet here we are as a nation with thousands of people walking around with type 2 diabetes or as pre-diabetic, because they would much rather sit with a bag of chips or bowl of ice cream and binge Netflix than take a stroll around the neighborhood after eating a bowl of berries. By the way, you can add some whipped cream and dark chocolate chips to your bowl of berries to make them more fun.

Fun, that is what we believe food is. We use food to celebrate birthdays and holidays and vacations. We fill our bodies with sugar and the wrong carbs and processed foods all for the sake of fun. Look, I love me some chocolate cake from Portillos in Chicago. I also love some Yardley Water Ice from Yardley, PA. But I don't eat them all the time. I believe in the 80/20 theory when it comes to food. The 80/20 theory means 80% of what you eat out of the day should be clean foods. Clean food would be fruits, veggies, nuts, fish, and poultry. 20% of the day you can enjoy fun foods like whipped cream on your berries, a small bag of Doritos with your turkey chili, or the serving size of a piece of cake or cookies. I also believe there are no "good foods" or "bad foods", however I do believe there are healthy and unhealthy foods.

Healthy foods fuel and heal your body. Unhealthy foods lower your energy and could potentially cause damage to your body if you abuse them. Unfortunately, most unhealthy foods are designed to make you addicted to them. Food scientists design additives to increase your desire for them and cause cravings. That is why unhealthy foods taste so freaking good! I don't believe if you eat some chips with your tuna fish sandwich once in a while you are going to cause damage to your body. However, if you have a habit of eating chips every day, especially if you are someone who carries the whole bag with you to the couch, then you're just asking for weight gain and high blood pressure.

The reason I don't believe in good foods vs. bad foods is because, as a society, we have conditioned ourselves to shame ourselves for eating "bad" foods. That, my friend, is really just a mind fuck. As women, we emotionally beat ourselves up for eating a burger or cookies. Again there is nothing wrong with eating those things AS LONG AS you are eating healthier food as well.

Here is an example from my own life. I know I will be eating a burger for dinner so for breakfast I will eat an egg white omelet filled with veggies and feta cheese and for lunch I will eat salmon or chicken with veggies or a salad with tuna. Alongside my burger I will have some roasted potatoes and a salad. What

I am doing here is giving myself the pleasure of eating the burger, which isn't necessarily the healthiest option of protein for me, but I am choosing side dishes that will have fiber and will be easier to digest. This is a balancing act within my meals that my nutritionist has taught me. It took some time to figure out how to enjoy my favorite "unhealthier" foods without beating myself up thinking I ate "bad" food. Also, by balancing the unhealthier food with healthy options on the side, when I eat those types of foods I don't typically walk away feeling bloated and just gross. I enjoyed my burger and my belly still feels fantastic. It's a win/win.

One of the best rituals I have created when it comes to eating food, especially if I am faced with eating something that is not healthy, is asking myself before I eat it, "Is this food helpful or hurtful to my body?" Knowing if the food is or isn't going to help my body, meaning giving me energy instead of making me feel bloated and sluggish usually will help me to decide to choose a healthier food option over an unhealthy food option. Also, asking myself that question makes me pause for a moment and really think about what I am about to do. I am also showing myself love and compassion because I am honoring my desire to eat the food, but I am also honoring my desire to treat myself well. If I am still struggling with the decision to eat the food then I use a ritual called "Body Talk".

BODY TALK:

- Take a few deep breaths inhaling and exhaling out of your nose and then return to your regular breath.

- Place your hand on your chest and if you can close your eyes.

- Release any thoughts in your head and imagine yourself eating the food.

- Eventually you will either energetically feel a pull in the front of your body or the back of your body and you will begin to literally lean forward or backwards.

- If you feel your body energetically pull in the back of your body or you are leaning backwards your body is telling you not to eat the food.

- If your body energetically feels like you are being pulled forward or your body is leaning forward then you know your body is acknowledging to eat the food.

Our bodies speak to us all the time! When we can take a moment to calm our breath and calm our thoughts, we can really listen to what our bodies are trying to tell us. Our mind will play tricks on us but our bodies will be truthful and honest.

I am all about mindful eating, meaning I am very intentional on what I eat and how I eat. Portion control is everything when it comes to mindful eating, whether you're eating healthy or unhealthy food. I look at portion control as creating boundaries around my food. We all know it's easy to eat too much unhealthy food in one sitting, but it is also possible to eat too much healthy food in one sitting as well. I don't count calories, but I do pay attention to the caloric intake of my food. For example, avocados are good for you, but unless that avocado is the bulk of my meal, I will only eat a quarter or a half of the avocado in addition to whatever else is in my meal, because I know that avocados are high in calories. When I do eat anything that is processed like Wheat Thins for example, with my hummus, I will check the serving size on the box and put the Wheat Thins on a plate and put the box back in the cabinet.

A great habit hack when eating a snack is to always put your snack on a plate, in a bowl, or some sort of container and WALK AWAY from wherever you removed the food, whether it's the cabinet or the fridge. It is too easy to stand in front of the fridge or the cabinet shoveling food down your throat. When you mindfully place your food with intention onto a plate and measure out your food by gauging a healthy amount of food, you are being intentional about taking care of yourself. This is a form of self-love.

I personally do not believe in "diets" because, to be honest, I have tried a bunch of them and yes, I may have lost weight in the process, but the minute I stopped the diet I gained the weight right back, and then some. Sound familiar? I am pretty confident the same has happened to you as well. I remember standing in my kitchen one day as I was following a very popular program that was centered around weight loss and weight control. This was around the time I was really starting to understand about clean eating and how processed food that is marketed as fat free or sugar free is actually a chemical shit storm. My dear friend Connie, who was on her own health journey and became a certified nutritionist while battling breast cancer, had been explaining to me that when food companies take out natural ingredients of food like fat or sugar, they replace those things with some sort of chemical. The food companies also put in certain types of chemicals that not only make the foods taste desirable, but the chemicals are also created so that we become addicted to them.

While following a particular program one time when I was in my "dieting phase," I was eating a lot of sugar free and fat free products, because they were "lower points". After Connie had shown me the light on the chemical shit storm I was eating that could cause cancer, I made a promise to myself to be very mindful of not purchasing those types of food products anymore. The hardest thing for me to give up was Diet Coke. It wasn't until Connie had lost her battle to cancer and gained her angel wings did I finally give up drinking Diet Coke on a daily basis. Diet Coke was the one thing Connie would insist I give up if I was going to give up any type of chemical shit storm food product.

With all that being said, I don't believe in diets, but I do believe in nutritionists. A nutritionist is a certified and trained professional who knows and understands the medicinal side of food. They can create a meal plan that works best for you especially if certain foods are contributing to your health in a negative way. The truth is foods that work best for my body are not the foods that are going to work best for yours. A nutritionist can figure that out for you. Diets are designed for masses of people, not specifically for you. That's why people have such a difficult time with losing weight and keeping the weight off.

Again, I want to make sure you understand the topic of weight doesn't have to do with you being a certain size. You know when YOUR body is not at its best and you know what range YOUR body should be weight-wise. That's another reason I don't believe in diets. Typically diets lump people at a certain height to be a certain weight, which I call bullshit. You and I may be the same height, but you may have a heavier bone structure than me or more muscle mass than me, so naturally you are going to weigh more. It is so important to have this discussion because I don't know a single person who doesn't have body image issues around their weight. Either we are chasing the weight of a celebrity or fitness guru or we are chasing the weight we were years ago.

The way we should look at weight is not by what the scale says but instead by our health. Is your weight affecting your health, meaning is your body swollen all the time, do you have high blood pressure, do you have aches and pains in your joints, or do you have difficulty walking up a flight of steps? If the answer is yes to these then it's time to talk to a nutritionist. I have great news for you. Most insurance companies will cover a nutritionist especially if you have underlying health issues. A nutritionist will work with you to find the right foods that are good for YOU by creating meals and menus with you that are beneficial to your body, not only so that you can lose weight but also achieve optimal health.

When Connie passed away, it was within days of my aunt unexpectedly losing her life as well. I was extremely close to my aunt while growing up and although she was my father's sister, she was extremely close to my mom, and ironically she worked with my friend Connie. Their passing was only months after I had lost my mother. Having lost three women who meant so much to me within months and then days of each other put me on an emotional rollercoaster for months following. I allowed my emotions to get the best of me and dropped my guard around my boundaries on my food for a while.

I would like to mention here that falling off your daily self-care routine can be a normal process when you are dealing with something so heavy like grief. We all saw it happen during the pandemic when everyone began to eat and drink more to numb the pain of dealing with the lockdown. When you have a daily self-care practice, you are very aware of when you are falling off your daily self-care routine, because you have self awareness of what you are doing. Not once in those moments of drinking the diet coke or eating more fun food or even consuming more alcohol than normal, while I was grieving, did I shame myself. I acknowledged what I was doing in the moment. I was doing it and gave myself grace. See that is the thing. I knew what I was doing thanks to my self-care routine. Then when I was at the point of knowing I was ready to jump back into my physical self-care routine of eating healthier, I also acknowledged I was going through some extreme emotional trauma and I knew I needed some assistance. I reached out for help and I hired a new nutritionist since my friend Connie was no longer there to guide me.

How did I know it was time to jump back into my physical self-care routine and eat healthier? Great question. I listened to my intuition, which I believe is our spirit guides whispering to us. Every time I would reach for an unhealthy version of food I would hear a whisper in my head, "That's not a good idea." Eventually the whispers became more frequent and were no longer whispers. They were a lot louder and more stern. I also was feeling and seeing a change in my body. My clothes were tighter, my skin was dry, I had dark circles under my eyes, and my energy level was non-existent. My nutritionist helped guide me back to my way of clean eating while allowing myself to still indulge in a healthy way of fun foods.

Within a few weeks my bloat was gone, my skin looked better, and I had energy to chase my grandsons around while playing with them. I do occasionally have Diet Coke when I am out somewhere. For example, if I am at the movie theater I will purchase a Diet Coke with my popcorn. However, I do not keep Diet Coke in my house, because if I do I know that is all I will drink. Allowing myself to have Diet Coke once in a while still fills my desire to drink Diet Coke but also keeps me from drinking it daily.

While I would "diet" in the past, I always found myself thinking about food all the time. I also found myself shaming myself when I indulged in a fun food, aka what society considers a bad food. I feel as though diets send the wrong message to people: food is bad and food is punishment. I don't want to emotionally beat myself up because I drank a Diet Coke or I ate an Oreo. I also don't want to binge eat a bag of Oreos because my emotions have gotten the best of me.

This is why having a daily self-care routine that caters to the five parts of self so that you are aligned in mind, body, and spirit is so important. I have found that if your emotions are not intact then most likely your nutrition won't be either. One tool a nutritionist may give you to use is to write a food journal where you log in the foods you eat for the duration of the day. Not only will you log in the food you eat, but you will also log in how you are feeling emotionally and physically at the moment you eat the food and then again an hour later. Typically, you would log your food journal for a week and then you will go back and look for patterns. Maybe you'll find that raw veggies are not a good match for your digestive system or maybe you'll find that you reach for sugar to numb emotion or maybe you'll find that you start off eating well in the beginning of the day but at night you make poorer food choices. It was through my food journal I realized how all of those things affected me, but most of all how addicted I am to sugar and how I turn to sugar to numb my emotions, good or bad.

I truly believe if you choose to make healthier food choices you will begin to see a difference not only in your body but also in your emotional and mental state, because the foods can affect you emotionally and mentally. When you choose healthier food choices you will most likely have more focus and clarity. You may also have less hormonal swings because foods can affect your hormones. Your emotional outbursts may lessen because you won't be experiencing sugar level crashes. And as I said before, food is medicinal, so if you eat healthier foods your immune system will become stronger and you will be able to fight off those nasty germs easier.

To sum up nutrition, eat more healthy foods throughout the

day. Here are suggestions on how to eat healthier:

- Eat more fruits, veggies, poultry, and fish.

- Avoid fried and processed foods as much as possible.

- Hire a nutritionist to help you create meals and menus that are best for your body, especially if you have an underlying health condition. Check your health insurance. They may cover a nutritionist.

- Stop looking at food as good and bad; rather look at food as healthy and unhealthy.

- Before you eat something ask yourself, is this going to help my body or hurt my body? But by all means enjoy your favorite foods from time to time.

- Use portion control and be mindful while eating.

- Use tools like Body Talk, a food journal, or listen to your intuition.

- Give yourself grace if you are going through a difficult time and just try your best.

SLEEP:

For me one of the most difficult parts of my self-care practice is getting enough sleep. I am one of those people who loves to get the most out of my day. For years, I would stay up super late to get all the things done whether that was cleaning or writing papers, when I decided to go back to college in my late 30s to finish my teaching degree. I literally would use the phrase "sleep is for pussies". I don't know why I thought I was a hard ass because I didn't sleep. I used to run on 4-5 hours of sleep. If I got a solid five hours, then I typically could manage to get through the day as long as I stayed in motion. If I sat down though, it was lights out. I didn't realize the damage I was doing to my body and my brain by not sleeping.

Just like everyone's nutrition is different, so is the amount of sleep people need. On average you should be getting 6-8 hours of sleep at night to ensure optimal brain and body health. Did you know it is just as dangerous to get behind the wheel of a car exhausted as it is to be behind the wheel of a car intoxicated? When we don't get enough sleep, our brains don't function well. We have brain fog, we can't focus, and we forget things. Mamas you know exactly what I'm talking about. Just think back to those first few months of bringing your new baby home and all of that sleep deprivation. I'm exhausted just from the memories.

Here is the mind blowing thing that I learned about sleep that changed my whole outlook on it. When we first fall asleep we are in what is considered a light sleep for about the first four hours of our slumber. Once we hit around the four hour mark that is when we fall into a deeper sleep. This is when all the magic begins to happen. During those hours our body begins to repair, rejuvenate, and fight off illnesses. This is why when we are sick, it is important to get sleep and why when we don't get enough sleep we are constantly sick.

Sleep also gives us energy to get through our day. Some days we may need more sleep than others and we feel like we need to nap. Naps for adults are great as long as they are for a short period of time. A nap mid-afternoon, unless you are sick, should be no more than 10-20 minutes. Once you get past 20 minutes you are beginning a whole new sleep realm and when you wake up you are groggy, because your brain has a hard time processing it is not bedtime. The same thing goes for hitting your snooze button on your alarm. Once you hit that snooze button you begin to drift off and start a whole new sleep realm. You think you are doing yourself a favor by giving yourself a few more minutes, but in reality your brain and body will function much better if you just hit that alarm off and get your ass out of bed.

For the longest time I wouldn't nap and for two reasons. The first reason being that when I would nap, I would nap way too long and I would wake up feeling like shit. My head would be in a fog for the rest of the day and then, even though I could fall asleep at night, I would wake up in the middle of the night and not be able to fall back to sleep. The other reason I wouldn't nap is because my mom was clinically depressed. I can remember her napping a lot, especially when I was a teenager. However, when I was in my early twenties my mom spent months on the couch either sleeping and crying and I was petrified that if I laid down for a nap I would wake up like her. I know now that would not happen, but at the time it was so awful to witness. Luckily my mom was able to work with doctors and eventually she got off the couch, but that trauma still sticks with me. If I do decide to close my eyes in the middle of the day for 10-20 minutes, I still sometimes have to have an inner dialogue with myself that I am not my mom. On days when I feel I need to close my eyes for a bit, which doesn't happen often, I set an alarm on my apple watch or my Iphone to make sure I don't sleep past 20 minutes. I always feel refreshed after my nap.

I never have trouble falling asleep. It drives my husband nuts. We can be anywhere and my head hits the pillow and I'm out cold within minutes. For the majority of my life, I have been able to sleep through the night, but I have noticed on days that I don't move my body or wasn't stimulating my brain during the day are the nights that I have trouble sleeping through the night. Prior to the pandemic I moved all day every day and my brain was constantly going as well. I slept like a rock. When the pandemic hit, that changed. It took me a while to realize that not moving my body or engaging my brain like I used to was affecting my sleep. I was no longer walking in and out of the school building or back and forth to my car at stores. Even though I was still working remotely I wasn't engaging in conversation with my co-workers and students like I normally did. I wasn't holding conversations with friends and family. I began to incorporate walking around the neighborhood every single day so that I was moving my body. I would listen to podcasts or audio books so my brain was engaged. Then, I began to sleep much better.

Now for all you new mamas, I know sleep is a totally different topic for you. My biggest advice for you is to sleep when you can get it. Let someone hold or feed your baby while you rest. I promise you baby will be okay and you both will benefit from you being more alert. I can remember those times pacing in my living room holding my babies who were completely content, but I was a blubbering mess because I was so sleep deprived. It's okay to ask for help so that you can take care of yourself so you are a better mama. I also promise that the season of sleep deprivation will pass. You will once again get sleep by learning to adapt to the sleep schedule of your children and maybe hopefully you will be blessed with those unicorn children who like to sleep in. Unfortunately, I never experienced that, but from one mama to another, I wish that experience for you.

For those of you who like to sleep in on the weekends I have some sad news for you. You can't bank hours of sleep by making up for not sleeping all week and then sleeping in all day on Saturday. It doesn't work that way. You need consistent sleep every night to live a healthy and happy lifestyle. I get it, you have a busy lifestyle. I totally understand that, but you won't be able to keep up with that busy lifestyle if you don't get your rest.

I already shared that moving your body and engaging your brain throughout the day will help you sleep better. Another ritual I do when I get into bed is practicing scanning meditation. I have practiced this meditation for most of my life and I learned this meditation from my French teacher in middle school. She would have us enter her class room, instruct us to sit on our desks, and she would lead us in a meditation so that we would release all our emotional and mental crappy energy, and she would have our full attention and focus. I literally don't remember how to speak French now, but I took away two amazing learnings from her classroom. One, french fries do not come from France and two, how to meditate. At bedtime my meditation practice has become so ingrained as a habit for me that I don't even have to think about doing it. I just automatically start scanning my body. I take a deep inhale through my nose and exhale out of my mouth. I imagine a warm bright light over my head. The light touches the top of my head and then I imagine feeling the warmth of the light on the top of my head. I then allow the warm bright light to drip over my forehead, relaxing my forehead, then continue to drip down the back of my head, then over my temples, and then my eyes. I allow this light to drip all the way down each area of my body all the way to my toes focusing on each area of my body as the light hits it to release and relax any tension. If I haven't fallen asleep by the time I get to my toe, which typically I have, I then release the light starting at the top of my head and ending with my toes.

This is by far one of my absolute favorite meditations and is a wonderful tool to create a ritual around your bedtime. I have practiced scanning meditations countless times over my life and not just at bedtime. I practiced this meditation when I was in labor with my kids to help relax my body and my mind. I would also practice this scanning meditation when I was sitting in waiting rooms at the ER when my mom was being admitted into the hospital and when I was sitting in the cardiac waiting area of the hospital while my husband was in surgery after he had a heart attack. I love this meditation so much that when I was teaching mindfulness classes to school staff members, I would incorporate this meditation into my mindfulness lessons. Today I share the scanning meditation with all of my yoga students and we practice the scanning meditation at the beginning of every class.

I know that life is busy and life is hard and that it can be difficult at times to sleep. Some nights you are up worrying about your to-do list the next day or maybe your teenager just got their driver's license and you lay awake at night conjuring up the worst scenarios in your head, or maybe you have childhood trauma that makes you afraid to fall asleep. I know for a lot of people the quick fix is to grab sleeping pills and yeah maybe they help you fall asleep. However, they are never a healthy solution to not sleeping and highly addictive, especially prescription sleeping pills. I watched what sleeping pill addiction looks like with my mother and it was unsettling.

There are so many ways to naturally fall asleep and I will share tips and tools and rituals I have used to get some sleep. Obviously the first one is the scanning meditation but there are so many other meditations you can do to aid with sleep, especially guided meditations. Guided meditations are readily available for you at all times and for free thanks to Google and YouTube. I enjoy the Calm app, but regardless, there are thousands of guided meditations out there that are specifically geared towards sleep. You can either meditate before bedtime or get yourself comfy in your bed as you melt into your bed during your guided meditation. Guided meditations will help relax your mind along with your body, as it settles down your heart rate and nervous system.

Another tool I use to get some sleep is to diffuse lavender oil in my bedroom. I put the diffuser on about an hour before I go to bed so that the room smells delightful and serene. Lavender oil promotes relaxation which can improve sleep quality for those who suffer from insomnia, depression, and anxiety. It is one of my absolute favorite essential oils! Diffusing the essential oil is a part of my night time ritual, or routine if you don't vibe with that word. Some nights I even take a warm bath with Epsom salts and lavender oil. Between the warmth of the water, the Epsom salts, and the lavender oil, my body feels so relaxed I head straight to bed.

On the nights I don't take a bath, especially the cool nights here in New Jersey, I like to take a dip into our hot tub. After one cycle of the hot water and the jets I am ready to put my head on my pillow. In the evening about an hour or two before I go to bed, I turn off all the bright lights in my house. I make a conscious effort not to look at screens including my phone. Blue light has an effect on our brains and keeps them active. We want to quiet our brains down before bed. I do however watch television, but I will only watch lighthearted and funny types of shows and movies. Friends is my bedtime friend. I go to bed every night with Friends on my television because it is comforting, it makes me laugh, and it makes me feel a sense of security. Most nights I don't even watch an entire episode. It's just something about listening to my Friends at Central Perk makes me feel comfy and relaxed.

I started this ritual of Friends a few years ago. My husband would always want to put the news on to watch the weather before bed but the news is the news, violent and negative. At that time everything, including the weather, was becoming accessible on the phone. I asked him if he really needed to know the weather before bed, which never changed from the

5:00 news weather predictions, and to find the information elsewhere like on his phone. Eventually he stopped looking at the weather at night because he realized the weather didn't change, unless a snow storm was brewing. What he had created was a habit of watching the news for the weather and over time he changed that habit.

Let me side note here again. Our lives are created by the habits we create. How we live our lives is determined by the choices we make to do things. It starts off by doing something once and then doing it again and then again and again. You know where I am going with this. When we find ourselves in a season of life and we are not feeling fulfilled or getting results that we want we need to ask ourselves what are the habits that we have created that are stopping us from creating the life we want. Is the glass or two of red wine after dinner stopping you from getting up in the morning to work out so that you can have the fit and healthy body you want, because your head is in a fog? Is the habit of binge watching Netflix preventing you from working on the project you have been dreaming of doing?

Once you recognize the habit you need to change, you then need to figure out what habit you can replace it with. Then start implementing that habit. In my experience this will go one of two ways. Either it will go smoothly and transition well. I love when that happens. But, if you start to find resistance to that habit, you must start asking yourself this question, "Why is changing this habit so hard?" Maybe you feel you NEED those glasses of wine at night. Spoiler alert, you don't NEED those glasses to wind down. You have created a habit of THINKING you need those glasses of wine to wind down. Maybe you love the ritual of holding something in your hand at night. Great, change what is in your hand. Change the wine to a cup of tea. Chamomile tea that is very relaxing to drink at night. Every time I drink it I feel just as relaxed as if I drank a glass of wine and have no foggy brain in the morning!

To sum up, a nighttime ritual or routine will set you up for success for a good night's sleep.

- Turn off the screens at least an hour before you go to bed. If you have to use screens before bed, use blue light glasses while you are using them.

- Turn down the lights in your home about an hour before bed.

- Diffuse lavender oil or burn a lavender candle so that the aroma in your house is relaxing and serene.

- Take a nice warm bath with some Epsom salts and lavender oil to relax those muscles and your mind.

- Get a restful night of sleep with the amount of hours that work best for you that allows you to function.

- If you are constantly battling with your immune system, have brain fog, or feel exhausted throughout the day, adjust your bedtime routine to going to bed earlier or setting your alarm clock later.

Taking care of yourself through movement, hydration, sleep and nutrition is the base of the foundation that you need to live a healthy and happy lifestyle. Think of your physical self as your floor. It's where you stand up and what keeps you steady. A healthy functioning body will create happiness in your life. You will have the freedom to enjoy more things in life and will have the energy to enjoy them.

I have seen what an unhealthy body looks like with my mom. Her unhealthy body led her to depression, anxiety, addiction to sleeping pills and cigarettes. She disassociated herself from the world because she was embarrassed about her appearance. My mother aged about 20 years in a matter of 5 years. She was a vibrant beautiful woman who never left the house without her hair done and even her dress down clothes were fancy. She visited the dentist not twice but three times a year. About four years before she passed, I sat in the waiting room of a dental center as she had multiple teeth pulled and was fitted for dentures.

An unhealthy body leads not only to disease of the body, but also to the mind. She suffered from diabetic brain which often resembled Alzheimer's and dementia. An unhealthy body leads to losing your freedom. One of the most difficult decisions my sister and I had to make was to take away her ability to drive her vehicle after she put her phone in the microwave instead of her oatmeal and blew it up. There were a few other incidents as well where she was passing out. After her dialysis treatment, she would like to drive herself to get lunch. She passed out in the Chinese food restaurant and when the ambulance arrived, she refused to get in the ambulance. One time my son picked her up from dialysis and my mom wanted a cheeseburger from

McDonald's. Do you see the trend here of unhealthy eating? While they were in the drive-through my mother passed out and slumped over. My poor son still carries that trauma with him. He will jokingly say, "Remember that time I thought MeMom died in my truck?" But at the time isn't wasn't a joke or funny.

We watched my mom deteriorate in front of our eyes. She saw it too. I can remember one day sitting in her hospital room and she picked up her arm. Her skin was just hanging from her bone. There was no muscle. She flicked at the skin with her fingers and said, "Look at this skin hanging; it's disgusting". Or the time she looked in the mirror and you could tell she was sad by her reflection. She sighed an audible sigh and said, "I look like an old hag."

As I type these words tears are stinging my eyes and rolling down my cheeks because I know behind that saggy and wrinkled skin used to be a vibrant woman who loved to laugh all the time. She was always the dancing queen at weddings and parties. My kids always knew when their MeMom arrived for a visit because you could hear *NSYNC, Bruno Mars, or the Pussycat Dolls blasting from the speakers of her vehicle. My mom always said, "Music was meant to be played loud so if you are ever expecting me at your home you'll know when I arrived by the tunes coming out the speakers of my vehicle."

I know that there are times when people become unhealthy and it has absolutely nothing to do with their lifestyle. My husband had a heart attack in his late 40s. At the time he was working out regularly and we were eating extremely healthy. The only downfall for his health at the time is he is a tobacco dipper. So gross, right?

I'll never forget. We were in NYC in MoMA and he clenched his chest and turned completely gray. The days and weeks to follow were extremely emotional and stressful. By all means my husband should not be alive today. His heart attack was in the artery cardiologists referred to as the widow maker. Calcium had built up over time, and on that day a piece of the calcium broke off. Typically, the broken calcium creates a dam in the artery so that the blood can not flow. Most people drop dead at that moment. When my husband grasped his chest, he should have fallen to the ground and died. By the grace of God, he didn't. My husband did have surgery days following the heart attack and the robotic team was ready and on standby waiting because by the measure of my husband's calcium, they were expecting the worst. When my husband's cardiologist entered the waiting area, after only forty minutes instead of the hour or more he said it would probably take, my heart felt like it was going to stop. I thought the worst had happened. His cardiologist looked at me and said, "He's done; you can see him soon." I asked if he had bypass surgery and he replied no. I asked how many stents were put in and he replied none. I just looked at him stunned, and he looked back at me with the same bewildered look. He said, "I can't explain it other than your husband must have had angels by his side the day he had the heart attack." At my husband's follow up appointment, we learned that the cause of the calcium was his cholesterol level, however his cholesterol level had nothing to do with the way he was eating or moving his body. He could work out every day and eat the healthiest of foods, yet his body would still have a cholesterol issue. My husband now has to take medication for the cholesterol and that medication causes side effects, which in the beginning, were not fun.

Here's the thing though. If my husband would have gone to his annual physical with his primary doctor and had blood work taken, it would have most likely shown high cholesterol levels and the heart attack incident most likely would have never had happened. I used to beg and lecture him because he needed to see a primary annually. He would just blow me off and tell me it was unnecessary. If something was wrong, then he would see a doctor. That is what is fucked up about the mentality of this world we live in. Preventative actions to take care of your health can prevent situations like me having to witness my husband clenching his chest in MoMA. Preventative actions could have prevented my children from having to rush home from college during finals to be by their father's bedside while he was having heart surgery.

Eventually I gave in on the begging and lecturing to see his primary. This is a hard truth to swallow my friend. We can't make people do things so that they live a healthy and happy lifestyle. What you can do is lead by example and hope that they see your journey of a healthy and happy lifestyle and in turn begin to live their own journey of health and happiness. It's like that old saying, "You can lead a horse to water, but you can't make it drink." My husband doesn't miss his physical appointments anymore. He learned his lesson the hard way.

If there is anything I'd like you to take away about your physical self from this book, it is this: you right now have a choice to take care of your body. You right now can move your body, drink your water, eat healthier, and get your rest. You right now can make an appointment with your general practitioner and have routine blood work drawn. You are in control of your body right now, so please don't become like my mom and let your body control you.

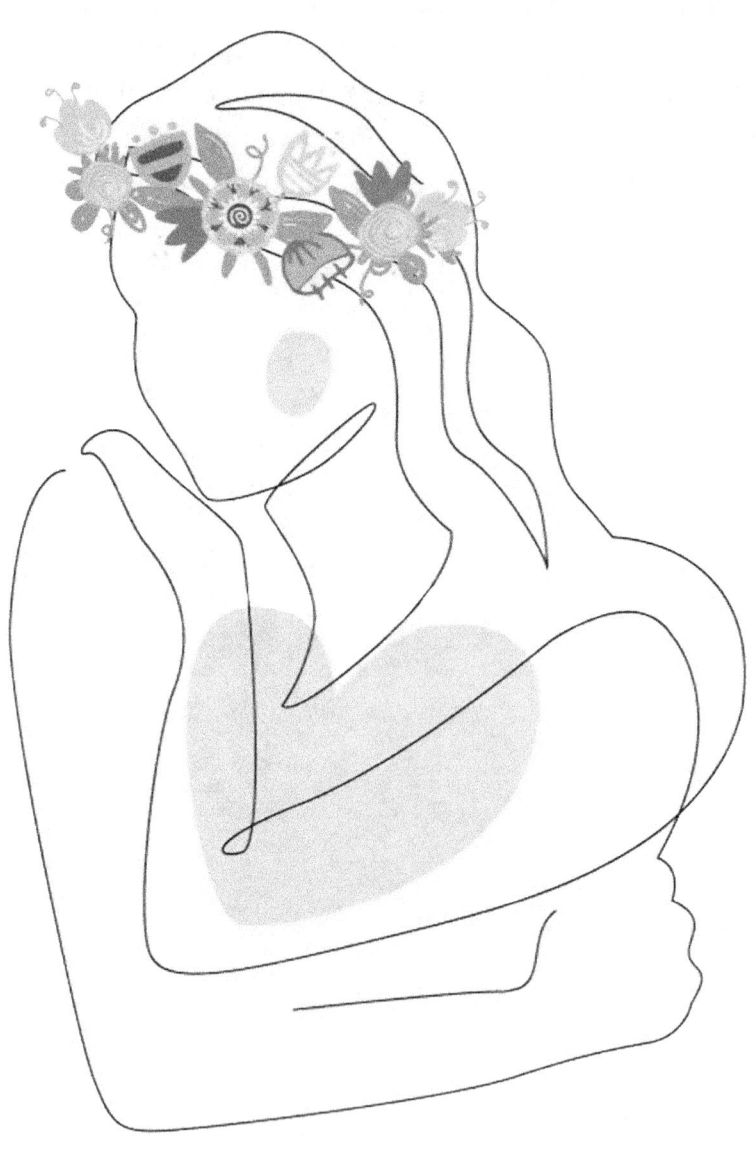

CHAPTER SIX

The Social Self

Social self-care is about cultivating a connection with other people. Those people consist of your friends, family or co-workers. Socializing with other people is so important for our mental health. Yes, even you, my introverted friend. If the last few years of the pandemic has taught us anything it is that as humans we are social beings. Not being able to interact with the people we love was excruciating to say the least. Not being able to hold conversations face to face or give one another a hug was devastating. It was wonderful that technology gave us the ability to not only talk to one another, but also to see each other through Face Time, Google Chats, and Zoom calls. I am truly grateful for those interactions; however, it's still not the same as being in someone's presence and feeling their energy while looking them in their eyes.

There is an exchange that happens between two people when they lock eyes and hold a conversation. It's knowing you each are present and not just hearing what the other person is saying, but listening as well. Yes, you can look into one another's eyes on a Zoom call, but something gets lost in the translation through the screen. I learned the hard way trying to teach six and seven year old children while long distance learning. I literally would have rather stuck a pen in my eye than have to talk to my students through a screen. Every part of my being as a teacher was dying inside every time I logged on. I am not saying distance learning doesn't work, because some people love it.

So much time was lost with loved ones during the pandemic and some of us even lost loved ones. I was fortunate when we placed my mom in hospice that at the time the world was opening up a little bit. I couldn't imagine how it would have played out if my sister and I wouldn't have been able to be there with her. I don't even want to think about it.

Just about everyone my mom loved and cared about was able to come visit her. If they weren't there in person, they Face Timed with her. She died after being showered with love by the people who loved her the most. Of course, there were the few people who trickled into the hospice center to say their goodbyes who barely interacted with her during the rough times while she was alive. My sister and I debated whether to allow them there because we knew their presence had nothing to do with our mother, but was more self serving. Same was for her funeral. There were people there I wouldn't dare talk to unless I had to. Having had a spiritual practice, I knew to look at them through the lens of love and not through anger, so we allowed them. I am glad we did, for my mom's sake. Now that she is gone, I will never have to deal with them again.

And I chose the route of distance learning to finish my teaching degree through University of Phoenix. At the time it wasn't the only option for me, but it was the best option for me. I was working at Parkway Elementary School in my home town. My title was "Security Monitor" and you may laugh at that title if you were to see me in person. I don't look the role of "security" at all! I am a petite 5'2" woman, but don't be fooled. That school was locked down as long as I was sitting at that front desk. However, often I was removed from the desk to cover teachers and paraprofessionals as a substitute.

What I loved the most was when a student was being transferred to our school district from their previous school district for a short time period. Typically, I was placed as their 1:1 para and I loved every minute of it. These students typically came from a rough home life, if they had a home life at all. At the time I didn't realize the tips and tools I was using were considered mindfulness. I just intuitively knew how to regulate their nervous systems through tools like breathwork or by finding the root cause of their breakdowns instead of reprimanding their behavior. I have always had the empathetic ability to look into someone's eyes and not only see but feel their pain. It is a gift and a curse.

Like most school districts who like to cut corners, my position was not a full time position. This way the school district did not have to offer me health insurance. So my position was 80% which worked well for me because I was able to get all three of my kids to school, and I was able to run home after work to do a few chores or errands before I had to pick them up.

All three of my kids were in their teenage years and attending middle school and high school. They each were very active in multiple sports, so in the evenings I was what we called in those days a taxi service. Now you young kids call it an Uber or Lyft service. I digress. At that time my husband was grinding at his career, making a name for himself and chasing his dream. Unfortunately, his dream consisted of him consistently being away from home most of the work week. He made it a rule for himself to always be home during the weekends. For years he spent one week out of the month at his company town home in California. The other weeks out of the month he split time between his office in the town next to our home town, Pennington, which was convenient. Most of the time he was flying all over the country at other work offices.

When he left that company to work for another, he began working in Manhattan which was a very long commute every day from our hometown in central New Jersey. That commute literally stole four hours of his day, every day, as he commuted back and forth to the city. Don't worry, he was still traveling with this company as well, only now he was venturing outside of the United States. I will give him a lot of credit despite all the traveling he did. He tried his best to be a present dad. He was still able to coach our son in baseball and football. He also coached our daughters' soccer teams. He never missed a sports game or a school function.

It was not easy and often a struggle not having my husband around. I took most of the grunt work at the homestead. But I know it wasn't easy for him to be away either. It was a sacrifice we both made in pursuit of the dream of bettering ourselves financially, greater than how we both grew up financially. We didn't grow up necessarily poor, but we weren't living in the rich side of town either. Yes of course, we wanted to buy our kids all the things like most parents do, but more than anything, we wanted to get them the fuck out of hometown to explore the world outside of our county. We wanted our kids to realize there is a life outside of our hometown.

Growing up, my husband and myself very rarely left New Jersey and if we did, it was a "vacation" to visit a relative. My husband and I both wanted our kids to see the world and to interact and socialize with people outside of our hometown. Loving your hometown is great! There is a lot of history and traditions and well, it is your home. However, it's very hard to evolve and grow when you are exposed to the same thing day in and day out. You need to broaden your horizons further than your county line in order to evolve and grow.

So back to my point of distance learning. I chose the route of distance learning to finish my college education to become a teacher because that was the best option for me at the time. Would I have loved to sit in a classroom filled with peers to bounce ideas off one another? Of course! But I was fortunate that during the day I worked with some of the most amazing teachers who I could bounce ideas off of and who also mentored me.

When the pandemic hit, there was no other choice but distance learning. Every educator I knew, especially in the primary grades, struggled just as much as I did. Not only were we struggling to make connections through the screen with our students but we were seeing things that, as educators, you never want to see in a student's home.

I bring all this up to say I worry for the children who were of preschool and primary grades during the pandemic. This is when children typically learn to socialize outside of their homes. This is when children start to interact with other adults other than family members or family friends and they create friendships with peers. When I talk to my former colleagues about the social skills these children have in the classrooms now that life has gone back to what I guess we will call "normal" after the pandemic, the consensus is unanimous and disturbing. The behaviors in schools are off the charts. The level of anxiety and defiance is at an all time high. My heart breaks for these babies. The trauma they have lived through during the pandemic will be carried with them for the rest of their lives. I pray and hope every day that we, as a society, continue having conversations about social, emotional, and mental well being not only for them but for all of us. I hope and pray that we continue to give them tips and tools such as creating a personal self-care routine so that they, too, can live a healthy and happy life.

Listen mamas, I am not just writing this book for you. I am

writing this book for your kids too. Remember what I said about leading a horse to the water? You can't make them drink the water, but if you model how to drink the water, they will follow your lead. Lead your kids to the water so that they can drink up. Show them how to have a healthy and happy life. Teach them how to build relationships and create space with other people while holding healthy boundaries. Teach them to be "me-ish".

So how do we have a healthy and happy social life? I'm so glad you asked that question. We begin by surrounding ourselves with people who lift us up, who inspire us, who motivate us, who comfort us, and who love us unconditionally. The number one way to live a negative shitty life is to surround yourself around negative shitty people. Misery loves company and misery is easy to live in because it is comfortable. Keep in mind, as I said before, comfortable doesn't always mean pleasurable. Comfortable means that something has become a habit. It is the norm. The longer you continue with the habit, the harder it is to break. Same goes for breaking the cycle of life long shitty friendships or the habits of finding new friendships or romantic relationships with toxic people. Those relationships are what we know and we fear changing those relationships. We are afraid of hurting their feelings or maybe we are afraid of what they and everyone else will think of us even though we know we should get out of those toxic relationships.

There is also the fear of the unknown if we let go and walk away. I can honestly tell you walking away can be uncomfortable. People will say things to you and about you. But do you know what? When you have peace and serenity in your life from being absent from all the bullshit you won't even know what other people are saying. You will be so busy living your best life. If by chance someone says something to you about you walking away from the toxicity, you won't even give a shit because you know what other people think of you doesn't matter. The only person's opinion about you that truly matters is your own. You don't need someone else's approval to establish boundaries and stay aligned to your principles about the life you want to live.

We are the culmination of the five people who we spend the most time with. The way you are living right now is a reflection of those five people. I have an exercise for you right now. Take out your journal or grab a piece of paper and write down the five people you spend the most time with. This includes family, friends, and co-workers. Next to their names write down how you feel around them and how they make you feel about yourself. Are they people who make you feel good about yourself? Do they not only hear you when you are talking, but do they really listen too? Are they there for you in the good and the bad times? Are they your biggest cheerleader when something great is happening in your life? Do they sit and hold your hand and wipe your tears on your worst days without judgment? If you answered yes to the majority or all of these questions, then that is a person you want to keep in your life. Now do you feel like shit about yourself every time you are around them? Do they only want to talk about themselves? Do they throw digs when you share good news about your life? Do they totally dismiss you when you are having a difficult time and judge you for being overly dramatic and tell you to get over it? If you answered yes to the majority or all of these questions, then that is a person you may want to let go of.

Now I know sometimes you can't completely let go of certain people who are toxic. You may work with these people or they may be family members you know you will have to interact with. These are the people you really need to create boundaries around. These are the people who will challenge you over and over again, but I promise once you start practicing boundaries with them, one of two things will happen. Either after time you will not give two shits what they say or do to you or over time they will realize that you will not fall into their toxic bullshit and leave you alone. That's the thing with toxic people. They have this fire burning in them to spread their toxicity. When you don't fuel that fire with your attention, that fire fizzles out.

Surrounding yourself around positive people as much as you possibly can encourages you to be positive. My favorite kind of people are people who are constantly smiling because smiles are contagious. I also love being around people who challenge me to be a better person and who encourage me to take risks. Your family and friends should love you unconditionally for your authentic self and without judgment. Can friends and family members offer suggestions to you about you? Absolutely! However, those suggestions should always come from a loving place, not a judgmental or controlling place. Their suggestions should be made with the intention to help you on your journey of being healthy and happy.

My dad always says that anyone you encounter in your life is there for a reason whether that encounter was for five seconds or lasts five months or five years or even a lifetime. Each person has a lesson and a purpose and is intended for a certain period of time. There will be people who you meet briefly and never see again. There will be people who are in your life for a season or maybe even a few seasons and then you drift apart. Sometimes those people will circle around but typically that relationship will never be the same as before. Then there are the lifers. The people who have been there since you were a kid or young adult. The ones who have seen you in your really good times and your really ugly times. They are the ones when you call and say, "I need help," and the only question they have is "How much bail money should I bring?" This is your tribe.

My tribe is very eclectic. Some of my friends are my actual family, like my twin sister who I have been friends with since the womb, and my cousin since she came out of my aunt's womb. Some of my friends I have had since elementary and middle school. We have grown up together and watched each other get married and become mamas. We may not see each other as much as we would like to, but we are always texting one another and are only a phone call away. When we do get together, we pick up as if we just saw each other yesterday.

Another group of friends I have I didn't become friends with until I was in my twenties. They are all the wives of my childhood neighborhood friends that I grew up with or as I like to refer to them, the boys from the hood. Did I mention growing up I was a tomboy? My twin sister liked to play with lip gloss and to stay indoors. I preferred fishing poles and being outdoors. My dad would take me and the boys from the hood to his hunting land to track deer or cut down trees. I will never forget the time a few of the guys came over to swim in our pool and my dad told us we had to take the roof of the house off first because he was replacing it. So, we climbed up with our shovels and started removing shingles from the roof before we jumped into the pool. I love that we are still connected after all of these years growing up together. Our friendship growing up brought me to their wives, who are now some of my closest girlfriends.

Then there are those friends of mine I met through my kids. You can become close to the mamas on the PTA and the soccer sidelines. You watch your babies grow and share the growing pains with one another. Typically what happens though is, as your kids grow up and grow apart from their friends, you grow apart from the parents you created friendships with. This isn't a bad thing and a lot of women I know get caught up in a lot of anger and sadness over this. This friendship was created by circumstance during a season of life. Seasons change. Your lives change. You are no longer hanging out at birthday parties together or scheduling carpool drop offs for soccer practice. Your friendships with those friends start to change when your kids start to become independent thanks to their driver's licenses. At this point you begin to find whether or not these friends were "seasonal" friends, because your interaction will begin to dwindle, and then the only encounters you will have will be when you run into one another at the Starbucks in Target or duck into another aisle to avoid talking to them. Not that I do that at all. Okay, maybe I do, but you know you do too. That is how you know that a friend is seasonal. You avoid them in the Target aisle. A lifer friend you run down the aisle to one another. There are those few gems from the parents of your kid's friend group that you remain friends with as your kids become adults. These friendships remain because they are people who you would have become friends with regardless of what season you were in or how you met. These friends become lifers.

The reason friends become and remain lifers is that they know friendship is a two way street. There is no pettiness between these two friends. They know that if they go days or weeks, or shit, even years without talking to one another, it's nothing personal. I see this with my clients often where they become bitter towards a friend, because they feel the friend hasn't reached out to them. My first question to them is, "Well what have you done to interact with them?" Usually the answer is "Nothing." To which I reply, "You do realize that friendship is a two way street, right? Maybe your friend is super busy or having a really hard time. I guarantee if you reach out to them, they will reply that they miss you and will fill you in on what has been going on in their life."

Don't just wait around for other people to reach out to you! Pick up the phone and call your tribe. Send them a "just thinking of you text" or meme that makes you think of them. It takes less than a minute to let someone know you are thinking of them.

Another thing we need to consider when it comes to our friendships is that our friends are their own unique persons and they give and receive love differently from one another and from us. When we learn how our friends give and receive love we no longer get upset when they don't react or respond the way we want them too. We know who they are as people and accept them for them. We also stop creating expectations around our friends. Some of my friends are introverted and would rather spend a night hanging out watching Netflix and drinking wine. Some of my friends like to be adventurous and jump on trains and planes to experience things. I respect my friends for the things they enjoy and the things they don't enjoy. I never push on them the things I want to do and they respect me in the same way. My besties also know that if we have plans and if one of them were to text me or call and say they need to reschedule I will always respond with "no worries". I don't need an explanation. I know how busy my friends are living their own lives and their lives with their families and other friends. Life is too short for petty bullshit.

One of the best ways to cultivate a friendship is to find like-minded people, especially like-minded people who are walking down the same path of a season of life. Like I mentioned before, the reason I was friends with the moms of my kids' friends is because in that season we were walking through life together as mamas of little people. We had a common lifestyle and common schedule, like dropping off and picking up our kids from school. Our kids had play dates together and attended school functions and played sports together. We literally would see each other almost every day out of the week. We forged strong friendships as we would talk to one another about all the things about raising our kids. We had that mama bond. As our kids grew, we grew, but eventually most of us grew apart.

It was beautiful to have someone to lean on and vent to and

celebrate mama moments with those who were going through the same season of life. It is so important for us socially to have other humans who understand what we are going through in life in real time. Today I rarely see my mama friends. I hold them dear in my heart and I miss those days, but I know today if I were to get together with them, we would reminisce, but as soon as the nostalgia wore off, we would realize we are all walking different paths now. They held space in my life at that time and I will forever love them for their sisterhood and their friendship.

We live multiple lives while we are here on earth. Think about your life when you were five years old, then ten years old, then fifteen years old, and so on. Your life at fifteen years old did not resemble anything like your life at five years old and neither will your relationships at those ages. I have watched so many people and have many clients who become so incredibly attached to another person and when they lose that person, whether it be from a break up or one of them moved away, or if there was unfortunately a death, that person feels as if their life has ended. Don't get me wrong. I totally understand there is a grieving process when we lose someone, especially when it comes to death. However, as my great Aunt Jean would say to me, "You can have a good cry but life moves on and so should you." I loved that woman.

Aunt Jean was one of the strongest women I ever met. I would drive past her house and there she would be, even in her 70s, pushing her lawn mower with her gardening gloves on wearing her Keds and rolled up denim pants and a bandana tied up in her hair. Although my favorite vision of her would be when I would drive past her house and she would be kneeling on her lawn cutting the edges of her grass down the driveway and sidewalk with scissors. She was a woman who wasn't afraid of hard work to get what she wanted out of life.

When I think about the idea we all live multiple lives during our lifetime I think about her. When my great uncle, her husband, passed away, she was on her own. She had to take care of herself and the house and although her kids were grown, she was on her own navigating as a single parent. A lot of women would have crumbled in her situation, but not Aunt Jean. Instead, she cried when she felt it necessary, wiped her tears, rolled up her denim jeans, laced up her Keds and mowed the lawn. I have no doubt Uncle John was looking down on her smiling. He probably also placed a dandelion in the lawn now and then to drive her crazy. He was a funny man.

I don't believe that when someone passes over to the other side that we need to let go of them. Instead, we learn to live with their physical absence. But I do believe that we need to let go of toxic people in our lives. Letting go of toxic people can be just as difficult as losing someone to death, because that person is still living and breathing and lingering around on this earth. There is also the possibility that you may need to interact with that person because they are a family member or co-worker.

Before we go any further on toxic people and relationships, I want to point out that I do not believe that because you have family blood running through your veins that you need to put up with ANYone's toxic bullshit. I don't care if the person is your mama, your daddy, your sister, your aunt, your uncle, your cousin, your niece, your nephew, or even your own child. Yes, I said even your own child. You are NOT obligated to be their punching bag or object of abuse whatever that abuse may be just because you are "family". I know I may get some backlash for saying that, but I wholeheartedly believe that family isn't blood. Family are the people who love you unconditionally, who hold space for you in the good times and the bad without expectations of what they can get in return from you for themselves. And family sure as fuck NEVER lays a hand on you inappropriately or beats you down mentally and emotionally.

The shit I saw growing up with my extended family still haunts me to this day. The fact that most of my family just swept a lot of it under the rug makes me sick to my stomach. Why some of them are not rotting away in jail today still baffles my brain. When my children were born, I made a solid promise to myself that my children would not be subjected to the shit I witnessed growing up, and for the most part, they didn't. There were times we had to interact with certain family members at weddings and funerals, but my kids still to this day don't even know who the majority of our family members are, because I chose to put up a boundary for myself and for them, so that they would not become a victim or be traumatized. I also should mention that I have over thirty first cousins.

My mom was one of nine children and my dad was one of four children. It is hard to keep everyone straight. Unfortunately, when my kids were in their teenage years, they saw a slight glimpse of my childhood as my two asinine uncles got into a fist fight on the front porch of the funeral home during my grandmother's funeral. I was mortified, but I also used the experience as a learning opportunity to explain to my kids as to why I held the boundary of not allowing those family members into our lives. Did I get backlash for not interacting with family members? You bet your ass I did, but the backlash felt a lot better than walking in and seeing my aunt's two front teeth missing, because my uncle punched her in the face.

I have a client who has created a boundary around family members who think that it is okay to put their hand out and ask for all the things without even a thank you in return. My client has lived most of life as a people pleaser. She was always the first person her family would call when they would have a melt down. She was always the first person they would call when they needed or wanted something and my client would oblige. However, whenever it came to my client needing or wanting anything, those family members were nowhere to be found. Those family members are the type of people, that as long as you are giving out things their hand is always out to take. The minute you stop giving, all of a sudden their hand along with the rest of them, disappear. That is, of course, until they need something again.

I taught that client how to build boundaries around those family members. My client no longer feels obligated to answer text messages or phone calls from those family members. Instead, she deletes their messages and goes on with her life. Does the situation bother my client? Of course it does. However, when my client receives any sort of interaction with those family members, I have taught her many different tools. First, do not respond right away. Our emotions always get the best of us so either we respond with an apology which there is no need for. It's just fueled by our fear of upsetting someone. Or we come in hot with anger. It is always best to pause for a moment and collect your thoughts and emotions before you respond.

Then I tell my clients they have one of two choices. They can either respond with a healthy mature response or they can not respond at all. A lot of times when we are dealing with people like my client's family members, they are very self-absorbed and narcissistic. Sometimes it is just better to protect your peace and not respond, than it is to add fuel to their fire.

I know what people say of me, especially family members, because other family members think they are doing me a favor by telling me what they say. Does it bother me sometimes? Of course it does. I am a human with emotions. Do I allow those emotions to get the best of me? Fuck, no. I allow those emotions to come in. I recognize where those feelings are in my body. I sit with the discomfort as I breathe through it, and I allow the discomfort to move through me until I feel it leave my body. Sometimes the emotions fade instantly and sometimes it takes awhile to get through it. If I feel that this person is still invading my energy and my thoughts, because that person keeps showing up either in my presence or in my thoughts, I practice cord cutting.

Never heard of cord cutting? Oh, my friend, this has been a valuable tool in my life and I want to share it with you.

Whenever we have an interaction with someone, there is an energy exchange between you and that person. This energy exchange causes an energetic tie between you and the person. We have energetic cords between people we talk to and deal with on a daily basis, like family and romantic partners and friends and co-workers. We also have energetic cords between the random person we smile at who held the door open somewhere for us. When we have an energetic cord with someone who is toxic, we want to cut the energetic cord that keeps us attached so that we can be released from their toxicity and no longer be tied to them.

When you want to cut a cord with someone, no matter what the reason is, the ritual is very simple. I do recommend when you do practice this ritual to center yourself in the way that you are not holding resentment and negative feelings to this person during the cord cutting. Remember we are trying to cultivate positivity into our lives. By cutting this cord, we are honoring our boundaries and acknowledging that this person is not someone who we desire in our lives in pursuit of a healthy and happy lifestyle. We choose to let them go.

CORD CUTTING:

- Close your eyes and take a few rounds of deep inhales and exhales.

- Visualize the person whom you want to cut cords with.

- Imagine the cord that is between you and this person. This cord can be attached to any part of your body to theirs.

- Tell the person who you are about to cut cords with that you are grateful for the lessons they have taught you in life, but you are no longer tied to them.

- Now imagine cutting that cord with whatever sharp object you chose to cut the cord.

- Once the cord is cut, visualize that person floating away from you until they disappear.

- Take a deep inhale and exhale and then blink open your eyes.

Cord cutting allows you to release any attachment you have to that person. But, the cool thing about cord cutting is you can cut cords with people who you love and still interact with and you don't have to let go of them forever. For example, if you are arguing with your mother because she is constantly pressuring you by guilt tripping you to do all the family holiday festivities, but you and your husband would rather lay on a sunny beach for a holiday or visit your in-laws, then cut a cord with your mother around her guilt tripping ways. Before you cut the cord tell her that you appreciate the love she has for you and that she wants to spend time with you especially around the holidays. Tell her that you love her, but you are an adult and you do not have to follow her demands on how to enjoy the holiday season. Then, cut the cord.

Now for those of you who are reading this and you are thinking what kind of woo woo shit is this? I want you to hear me out. Cord cutting rituals have existed for centuries. Yes, it does exist more in the spiritual realm of Self, but I want you to think of it as a baby being born. When a baby is in the womb, that baby is solely attached to their mother by a cord. When that baby is born and released out of the womb the cord is then cut. That baby no longer is solely dependent on their mama. This is what cord cutting does. It separates us from what we are attached to.

One of the biggest keys to living a healthy and happy lifestyle is surrounding yourself around the people who lift you up. There will be times that the people you love, whether they are family or friends, are going through a difficult time and may need to lean on you and that's okay. However, if you have someone in your life that is a constant Debbie Downer you may need to reevaluate that relationship and let them go. If you have someone in your life who is constantly ridiculing you, let them go! But those people who make you laugh and make you feel good to be around, who make you want to be an even better version of you and support you when you do, those are your people. And you have every right to pick and choose who your people will be.

So how do we create a social self-care routine? Once you find your people, make it a daily intention to keep a line of communication going with them. I have two friends in my tribe of people that I pretty much have contact with daily, whether it is through a text message or a phone call or sending reels on IG or a pic on SnapChat. These are my two go to's when I need to vent or need an honest opinion, because these two people have shown me time and time again that they are there to hug me in the hard times and in the good times. I recommend finding one or two people who you can have a similar relationship with to be in your tribe. I also recommend that these people not be your significant other. I do believe you should have a strong bond with your significant other, and that they are there for you at all times just like your friends. However, the bond you have with your friends and the bond you have with your significant other is totally different. When we add intimacy to a relationship, it brings the relationship to a whole different level. It's a level that only you and your significant other will have with one another. I mean, let's be honest, your husband does not want to hear or will understand your period woes.

One of the things that I am very intentional about when it comes to my friends is that I create friendship dates all the time with them. These friendship dates could be just grabbing a cup of coffee to catch up on our lives at a Starbucks or a dinner date at one of our favorite restaurants or taking a day trip to NYC to see a Broadway show. Just like anything else, friendships take work but the work should feel effortless. Yes, there will be times when your schedules may not line up and you may be playing tag/you're it with phone calls and texts to one another to set up a date, but putting in that kind of work to ensure you still see one another is worth that effort. Once you are together the time spent with one another should be so much fun that you laugh so hard tears run down your face. Or maybe you have such in depth conversations with one another sharing your thoughts, your fears, and your dreams that you walk away feeling like you owe your friend a co-pay for a therapy session. Friendships should fill your cup up, not deplete your cup.

Friendships should also be filled with unconditional love and understanding each other's love language. Love language isn't just for romantic relationships. Love language also allows us to understand our friends' wants and needs so that we can better communicate with them and enjoy each other's company.

There is an amazing book called The 5 Love Languages: The Secret to Love That Lasts, by Gary Chapman. I highly recommend reading this book for all of your relationships in life. Once you have an understanding of how other people receive and give love themselves, your relationships with everyone in your life will be astonishingly different. This book not only helped me in my relationship with my husband but even helped me with my relationships with my kids. Learning to understand how other people express their wants and needs in life and in love is a game changer. You will learn how to approach conversations differently so that you have a flow of communication with the people you love.

We also need to respect our friends' boundaries. For example, I have a very dear friend who doesn't like large crowds so I would never invite her to see a concert with me. Instead, I respect her boundary of not being in large crowds and our friendship dates are typically coffee shop dates or dinner dates.

I am also intentional in creating family dates whether that's with one family member at a time or a group of family members. Since our kids are now grown, my husband and I try to have family dinners once a week with our kids. Our rule is whomever can join in joins, but if you have other plans by all means don't cancel the plans or feel guilty for not joining us. By not putting an expectation on who is joining us, it leaves no room for anyone to become disappointed. I know my kids have their own lives and they also have significant others who have families of their own. Will I be sad if they can't join us? Of course, because I love my kids and their company. Will I be mad because they didn't come over on a Sunday during the summer to swim in the pool while we cook out on the grill? No! The intention is to love the time you have with your family (and friends) not to hijack all of their time.

Relationships are a two-way street. If you are missing your friend or family member, instead of getting your panties in a bunch because they are not reaching out to you, pick up the damn phone or drive over to their house and knock on their door. Life is too god damn short to be waiting around for other people, especially the people you love.

To sum up social self-care, be sure to surround yourself around positive and uplifting people. If you have people in your life that are not filling up your cup, reevaluate those relationships, and if need be, cut ties with them or at least cut cords with them. Create boundaries around your relationships with family and friends so that when you are with them you are not in danger physically, emotionally, or mentally. Be clear about your boundaries with your family and friends, but also respect your family's and friends' boundaries. Remember that we are all trying to just live our best lives and one way to do that is to not put expectations on ourselves and relationships. Relationships are a balance of being empathetic and compassionate without being a doormat to other people's wants and needs.

CHAPTER SEVEN

The Emotional Self

I do believe that if there is one area of Self that most of us struggle with it is the emotional self. How we react to our emotions pretty much determines how we live our lives. Did you catch what I said? <u>How</u> we react to our emotions. That's right, we have the ability to decide how we will react to our emotions. Emotional self-care allows us to become more in tune with our feelings.

What is the difference between an emotion and a feeling? An emotion comes first and manifests consciously or subconsciously while releasing emotion chemicals. As humans, we can experience up to 27 emotions. Then along comes our feelings which are experienced consciously after the emotion chemicals start to work in our bodies. Once we begin to feel the feelings, our mood is then determined. These feelings are sparked by an emotion and the feelings are shaped by our belief systems, personal experiences, and a thought that is linked with the particular emotion. In essence, the emotion causes a trigger.

Triggers can be negative, but they can also be positive. Unfortunately most of us don't pay attention to the positive triggers as much as we do to the negative triggers. For those of us who have experienced trauma in our lives, and I truly believe that we all have or will experience multiple traumas at some point in our lives, we are constantly living in a state of being triggered. When practicing emotional self-care, we learn how to check in with ourselves; we become more aware of our triggers; we notice our thought patterns good and bad, and most importantly learn how to work through our emotions, not around them.

Negative emotions and feelings can be one of the most uncomfortable things we experience. Our mind and our body are connected, so when we have an emotion that emotion can cause a physical sensation like a headache, backache, and stomach ache. If we don't get hold of those negative emotions and work through them, they can cause chronic stress which can lead to shortened lifespan. Chronic stress can upset your body's hormone balance, deplete your brain of chemicals required for you to be happy, and damage your immune system. I am convinced that chronic stress is what caused my mom to die at such a young age.

Negative emotions from trauma can stay trapped in our bodies, stored in our muscles and organs. Whenever we feel the negative emotion, the body sensation we felt as a result of the trauma resurfaces. What is causing the negative emotion at the moment may not resemble the original trauma, but your body remembers what it felt like. So, whenever you are triggered by that same emotion, your body reacts to it as if you are reliving that same moment. I don't believe that you can ever truly recover from the trauma, because it is now part of you. However, I do believe there are amazing tools out there to help us process through the emotions and we can take control of the emotion before it takes control of us.

The first thing I would highly recommend for anyone to do is to see a therapist. One thing that makes my heart happy right now about the current generation is that taking care of mental and emotional health is much more emphasized and widely acceptable than when I was growing up. It certainly was not acceptable when my parents were growing up and definitely not for their parents. When I was growing up if someone mentioned they were going to therapy they might as well have said they were put in a straight jacket and locked in a padded room. Today, as far as society is concerned, if you say you are seeing a therapist you'll most likely receive positive feedback.

I do believe if it is possible everyone should talk to a therapist when they can, even if they are not going through a difficult time or dealing with trauma. Talking to a therapist allows you to speak about all issues that you are dealing with. They help you process your thoughts and emotions. Therapy is also beneficial because you speak to someone who is removed from your life meaning they are not your family or friends or co-workers. A therapist will be unbiased. Whereas when you speak to a friend or a family member about a person or a situation, they are lovingly only going to tell you what they think is best for you or take your side to a situation. A therapist will look at the person you are having an issue with or the situation from all angles and will gently guide you into dealing with the situation in a way that you think is best for you. Not to mention, if you talk to your best girlfriends in a way that is really just venting about the douchey things your husband does, that is only going to make them think your husband is a douche.

I vividly remember my mom telling me when my husband and I were first married to be very careful of the things I shared with her about my husband, because she didn't want me to paint a picture of my husband in a way that she would be mad at him. With that being said, my mom meant sharing little stupid and petty argument things not if he was abusing me. But do you see the point I am trying to make here? Speaking to a therapist allows you to vent and deal with little annoyances that could maybe one day escalate into something bigger. A therapist will give you tools on how to handle your feelings when an emotion arises.

There are a multitude of types of therapy and therapists that you can speak to specifically to whatever situation or trauma you are going through. It also may take you a while to find the right therapist for you. Unless you have a resounding gut feeling about a therapist right away that the therapist isn't a right fit for you, I always recommend to my clients to give a new therapist a chance for a month or so. Then, if you feel you are not clicking, look for a new therapist. Also, keep in mind that you may work with a therapist for a long period of time but eventually that therapist may no longer be a therapist you need to be working with anymore. It is totally normal to outgrow your therapist. That is actually a good sign that you and the therapist have done the work!

I absolutely adore my last therapist. She was a godsend in my life! I originally sought her out to help me deal with the trauma around my mother's illnesses, her multiple trips to the ER, and hospital stays and rehab stays and blah, blah, blah. I began working with her in February of 2020 and was set to meet with her for the third visit when the world shut down. Thanks, Covid. We continued our therapy sessions virtually over the next two years. Thanks to her I was able to live through the pandemic with ITP and not lose my mind. Thanks to her I was able to teach the little people virtually and not lose my mind. Thanks to her I was able to live through my father being across the country while living through a pandemic and my step mother being diagnosed with colon cancer and not losing my mind. Thanks to her I was able to live through making the gut wrenching decision to place my mom into hospice and to watch her live out her last few days and ultimately take her last breath. She reminded me weekly to stay on top of my self-care routine so that I would stay grounded and focused on the important things and not lose myself in the anxiety and stupid dumb shit.

One of the best tools my therapist taught me was butterfly tapping. My therapist is trained in EMDR and during almost every session she would have me take some deep inhales and exhales and begin butterfly tapping with my eyes closed while she brought me back to traumatic memories. She would guide me to think back to memory and then allow whatever thoughts and feelings would come up. Sometimes those memories would take me right back to the trauma and other times those memories would lead me down a path of thoughts that had nothing to do with the initial memory, and then lead me to a new discovery of myself. I learned so much about myself during those sessions. Things I had no idea that had affected me from my childhood were, and still are, affecting me today. Memories I had shoved down deep inside so I wouldn't have to feel them, emerged.

Because of my therapist, I have a knowing of myself that I know I would have never unraveled without her. Generational patterns became visible and it became very clear the parts of me that needed to be healed. We would end our sessions with me returning to my safe space in my mind's eye using all of my senses while butterfly tapping. To this day I still use this tool when I am triggered and I share with my clients, and even my family and friends.

Before I started working with my therapist I wasn't a stranger to tapping. I have been using EFT, Emotional Freedom Technique, for years as a source to manage my emotions and thoughts. EFT tapping is a mind-body method in which you tap on acupuncture points on the hands, face, and body with your fingertips. As you tap you focus on the emotion and feeling you are hoping to resolve while you repeat a statement that will describe whatever the issue is at hand followed by a statement of self-acceptance. An example of an EFT statement would sound like, "Even though I feel anxious, I deeply and completely accept myself." or "Even though I don't feel loved by others, I deeply and completely love myself." There are many wonderful videos on YouTube that you can follow if you feel intuitively you would like to try this tool.

What I love about EFT is there is movement involved. As you know from my previous chapter on the physical self, I believe movement is so vitally important for not only our body but for our mind. Sometimes we need more than just a movement. When we are able to use our mind's eye to visualize what is evoking a feeling, then audibly speak a statement about that feeling followed up with a positive narrative, while kinesthetically tapping on acupuncture points, we are able to bust through blocks and barriers. Words are wands and what we say becomes our reality. One of the best quotes I ever heard about thoughts is from a certified psychiatrist named Dr. Amen. He has stated, "You don't need to believe every stupid thought you have." This was one of the best things he ever learned while in medical school. It changed the way he thought about thinking and it certainly has changed mine. We don't have to believe all the negative crap that goes on in our head. We can choose what it is we want to listen to in our head. All we need to do is to change the trajectory of our thinking.

Like I said, words are wands and that means whether they are spoken out loud or just thought inside your head, your words have power. Let's face it, we all have a negative reel that spins inside our heads. That negative reel is constantly filling our heads with bullshit thoughts about ourselves. Some of those thoughts are in our head because of traumatic experiences we have experienced. Or maybe the thought is because someone said something to us that was negative about us. We internalized their opinion as the truth, and continuously remind ourselves of their bullshit opinion that is not the truth. Or maybe we look at other people and compare ourselves to them creating the narrative that there is something wrong with us.

I need to tell you this right now, because I also need to hear this right now. There is nothing wrong with you. You, my friend, you were divinely put onto this earth to shine as who you are. There is only one you. This world needs you. I need you. I need you to help me guide this world with light and love. If you are reading this book right now, that is not a mistake. You have been called to my words not because I'm some kind of expert or guru or whatever, but because you just needed a little reminder that you are fucking awesome, scars and flaws and all.

What we feed our brain is just as important as what we feed our bodies. The minute you start feeding your brain shitty thoughts is the minute you will start to believe your shitty thoughts. The minute you feed your brain positive thoughts is the minute you will start to believe positive thoughts. Yes, it is that simple! However, you need to keep repeating those positive thoughts until they become a habit of thinking positively. This doesn't happen overnight, but I promise it will happen.

So how do we train our brain to think positive thoughts? First, we need to capture all the negative thoughts we have in our head. One tool I like to use to capture those negative thoughts is a brain dump journal. A brain dump journal captures your thoughts throughout the day and once you finish the journal you can go back to find your negative thought pattern.

How To Brain Dump Journal:

- Set a timer on your phone three times during the day; once in the morning, once in the afternoon, and once in the evening.

- When the timer goes off, set the timer again, but this time for one minute.

- Write down every thought you have in your head for that minute no matter what the thought is.

- Do this practice for at least 3-5 days.

- Once you have completed the days go back with a highlighter and highlight all the negative thoughts you have had and compile a list of the negative thoughts.

Some of those negative thoughts can sound like: "I'm so tired." "I'm so stupid." "I can never have that." Once you have awareness of your negative thoughts you will begin to notice them when they creep into your head. When the negative thought creeps in you will make a conscious effort to flip the narrative of your thought. For example, if your negative thought pattern is, "I'm so tired" your flip to that narrative would be "I feel tired, but I know I can get to bed early tonight." Or if your negative thought pattern is "I don't deserve this," your flip narrative would be, "I am a good person and I deserve nothing but what is best for me." This tool does take some time and a lot of practice, but like anything else, the more you practice this tool the more it will become a habit where eventually you won't even need to think about doing it. You will just do it.

Positive thoughts create positive feelings that can make us feel like we are on top of the world. Look, I am going to be very honest with you right now because we are friends. I am sure you are thinking right now, and if we were in a one-on-one client meeting you would ask me, "Am I going to feel positive all the time?" My answer would be…Fuck no! Shit happens. It's called life. There is negative stuff that we can't control that gets thrown at us all the time. We can not control the outside world, but we sure as hell can control our inside world. The more you practice positive thinking thoughts, the more positive your life will become for the majority of the time.

Once you have an awareness of your negative thought patterns, you can also use the tool of positive affirmations to add to your tool chest. A positive affirmation is a statement that can help train your brain to look for positivity, build you up, and improve your confidence. You can write your positive affirmation(s) in your journal each day or you can also write positive affirmations on a sticky note pad. After you have written the positive affirmation, read the affirmation out loud. Then place the sticky note on your bathroom window or on your refrigerator or the dashboard of your car or in your pocket, so that you can reference your positive affirmation throughout the day.

Here are some examples of positive affirmations:

- I believe in myself.

- I am worthy.

- I make the best of every situation.

- I am abundant.

- I matter.

- Good things are coming my way.

- I choose peace.

- I deserve to feel good.

Remember you have a choice in believing who you are and how you want to live your life. Don't let negative self-talk become your narrative that makes you believe you are something you are not. It is great when other people love us, but the person who we must be most concerned with loving us is ourselves. I don't mean loving ourselves in a selfish way where we become self-absorbed. I mean loving ourselves in a way where we show ourselves the same amount of love and compassion as we do to other people. I am sure you have people in your life who you love deeply who are battered and scarred, and you love them unconditionally. You love them despite their flaws and mistakes. Why can't you love yourself in the same way?

If you are struggling with self-love, and my guess is if you are still reading this book you are, another tool you can use is "mirror talk". This is going to sound like a super simple task, but trust me, it is not. You may feel uncomfortable, especially the first time you try it. I remember the first time I practiced mirror talk, I was a blubbering mess in the end. Now when I practice mirror talk, I walk away from the mirror smiling.

Mirror talk:

- Stand in front of a mirror.

- Set a timer for one minute.

- Look at yourself in the eyes.

- Repeat over and over to yourself "I love you".

The first few times you say I love you it will seem like no big deal. However, after some time you will begin to feel an emotion come up. You will begin to feel feelings. Thoughts will race through your head, and the more you say "I love you", the more uncomfortable you will begin to feel. Stick with the process and you'll begin to unravel thoughts and feelings that you've had about yourself. You will find a whole new awareness of who you are and you'll learn what parts you need to heal so that you can return to self-love.

We are accustomed to looking outside of ourselves for reassurance, acceptance, and for love. We compare ourselves to everyone, and these days, I mean everyone. Thanks to social media we have a sneak peek in people's lives. But that's the thing. It's just a peek. Social media has us believing that other people have the lives we want when the reality is people only share what they want other people to see, me included. Look, my entire life and your life does not need public knowledge. Yes, it's great to share accolades and even some of our struggles. It's great to catch up with old friends and to keep in touch with long distance relatives. But y'all, social media is not real life.

Let me say that again.

SOCIAL MEDIA IS NOT REAL LIFE! It's a tool you can use to socialize. That's it! Real life, that's hugging your friend when you see her at the coffee shop because you haven't seen her for weeks. Real life, that's running out the door at 11:30 at night after your sister calls you that the ambulance is on the way for your mom. Real life is when your kids ask when the next Sunday Funday pool day is going to be because they want to be with you. Real life is staying up until 3:00 in the morning to write a college term paper while your husband and kids sleep because that's the only time it's quiet in your house. Real life, that's when you gave up your entire weekend to grade report cards. Real life is when you lay on the floor next to your fur baby as the vet gives her a shot so she can cross the rainbow bridge. Real life is the dishes in the sink at 7:00 in the morning because you didn't have the energy to even put them in the dishwasher. Real life is messy and complicated for EVERYONE! Don't be fooled by the reels and the stories. They are filled with filters to make you believe they are something they are not.

For those of you who grew up before social media, like me, we still had comparison issues. We just compared ourselves in different ways. I can remember being in the gym locker room at high school and comparing my body to the other girls as we got changed into our gym clothes. I have always been vertically challenged and since puberty I have had curves. I hated my boobs since I started growing them when I was 11. I would hide them under baggy shirts or wear a jacket. I was ashamed of my body. Luckily for me, I was very much a tomboy, so I really didn't care much about fashion. Later in life, after a lot of therapy and healing, I realized I was hiding my body not out of shame, but because I had grown up around men who abused women, physically and sexually. I was hiding my body out of protection. I was never physically or sexually abused by anyone growing up. I thank my mom and dad for their protection. I did have one very creepy and disgusting encounter with one of my uncles one day, but because I had enough awareness of how deeply fucked up and mental he was, I was able to leave the conversation just feeling skeeved and not touched. The conversation was about my boobs, so needless to say, I became even more insecure about them.

Even though I was insecure about myself, I had enough security in myself to not allow someone to take advantage of me like that. There was no way in hell I was going to let a man do that to me.

My insecurities ran deeper than my boobs. I hated gym class because I hated that we would have to change into our gym clothes in front of other people. I would change my shirt and notice the other girls who had on tiny bras, but I also noticed the girls who had flat bellies and wished I looked like them. I felt ashamed of my body. Little did I know that later in life I would hold conversations with those girls as adults and find that they were just as insecure and ashamed of their bodies as I was. How fucked is that? When are we going to teach our daughters to love their physical self? That their body is beautiful as it is? It wasn't until I was older that I learned to love my body and learn the fact that God lovingly made me as I am. This vessel that my soul is being carried in was purposely created just for me. And guess what, I learned to love my boobs. I mean come on how cool is it that I got to feed my babies from my boobs?

Having an awareness of who we are is a superpower. It makes us a stronger person and allows us to make decisions about and for ourselves that serve us well. Part of having an awareness of who we are is also having an awareness of our own emotions. When we have an awareness of our emotions, we are better able to understand ourselves and the bonus is we are also able to understand other people's emotions as well.

One of the best tools out there to find awareness of our emotions is journaling. I have found one of the best ways to really learn about your emotions is to write a free flow journal. I particularly like to do free flow journaling first thing in the morning, but I have written in this journaling format at various times of the day. The reason I like the morning is because my brain is fresh and clear of a million thoughts I have gathered throughout the day. I begin writing whatever comes to my mind in my journal. It could be something as simple as I hear the birds chirping. My coffee is delicious. I just unconsciously write my thoughts for at least three pages. Some days my pen just flows and other days it's a struggle. However, on the days that my pen flows, typically I reveal something that has been bothering me, feelings I have kept bottled up, or I receive an a-ha moment. I will go from writing "my coffee is delicious" to "I can't believe that bitch said that about me!" and the pen just keeps going. The days my pen flows, typically the revealing moments happen on pages two or three. Once we clear out all the nonsense in our head it makes space for the important stuff to come forward. I tell my clients to try not giving up writing after page one, even if you feel stuck or you want to stop.

I feel that a free flow journal is sometimes better than talking to a friend or a therapist. You clear your mind of all the shit that is weighing you down. Purging out your thoughts and your emotions is therapeutic. There are so many benefits to this type of journaling. It allows you to see patterns of thoughts, positive or negative. You find a realization of where you may need boundaries. You uncover an awareness of where you may need to begin healing old wounds and traumas.

I also tell my clients not to be afraid to put their thoughts down on paper. Your journal is for you. Nobody else needs to read your journal unless you don't mind others reading your thoughts. Also if there is someone you are concerned about reading your journal without your consent, then you may want to reevaluate your relationship with that person. Your privacy should never be invaded in that way. If someone is invading your privacy, then that person definitely has some deep seeded issues of their own they need to deal with.

If there is something you need to write down that you absolutely do not want other people to read, even if you trust everyone around you, but you really don't want this information to be read for whatever reason, then I recommend creating a burning ritual after you write down what you need to put to paper. For some people this ritual helps deal with acknowledging past trauma and for others it may help with letting go of something. Once you are finished writing what it is you need to write, safely over a sink or a glass jar or a fireplace, light the paper and let that bitch burn. This ritual not only allows you to release your thoughts, but it also symbolizes to you that you have control over your thoughts and feelings.

While journaling, feelings will arise and they can be triggering. Just note that when you feel a feeling, you have control over that feeling. Allow that feeling to emerge. Use the heart hold in this moment. Sit with the feeling and feel the feeling giving it permission to be in your body. Notice where the feeling resides. Is it in your chest? Your belly? Your back? Talk to the feeling. Let the feeling know you are there with it and that the feeling is safe and you have control. Breathe deep inhales through your nose and release deep exhales out your mouth. If you need to, repeat over and over "In this moment I am safe". Once you feel the feeling begin to dissipate, thank the feeling for revealing to you what you need to feel and to heal. Then, let the feeling go.

Did you know that fear and excitement feel the same in the body? What happens in your body when you become excited? Your heart may start racing. Your belly may do flip flops. You may get sweaty or jittery? Now think about what happens in your body when fear arises. You get the same exact body sensation. I have a client who has had severe anxiety attacks so much in the last six months she has lost count on how many times she has been to the ER, because her heart starts racing, her belly does flip flops, and she starts shaking. She gets herself so worked up because she feels the body sensations and then her mind starts spiraling. She literally starts throwing up or has diarrhea. One of my coaching sessions with her I shared about how our body sensations are the same whether we are excited or scared. The body sensations are an indication that something more intensive is actually going on with her beyond her physical ailments. There is some deep rooted trauma or even traumas that she needs to work through with a therapist to help her reveal what it is and to work through it. Remember our bodies talk to us when our minds can't. You will start feeling things in your body long before you have an awareness about a thought that has popped into your head.

A great tool that I use for my clients and for myself to try to track what may be going on subconsciously when dealing with a physical issue is the book, "Heal Your Body" by Louise Hay. In her book, Louise Hay writes how when our body has a physical problem there is usually a mental probable cause and offers a metaphysical way to overcome the physical problem. Louise Hay believed, as I do, that the course of our words can create the outcome of our lives. The things we say of ourselves and to ourselves become our truth. She also believed that our thoughts contribute to whatever physical problem that we may be suffering with and if we change our words within our thoughts, we can change the physical problem. In the book "Heal Your Body," Hay lists problems with probable cause and provides a new thought pattern. For example, if your problem is indigestion then the probable cause could be gut-level fear, dread, or anxiety. The new thought pattern would be "I digest and assimilate all new experiences peacefully and joyously."

The next time you are experiencing indigestion and you obviously haven't eaten food or drank anything that would cause the indigestion, I want you to sit and listen to your thoughts. Pay attention to what is going on in your brain. Try free flow journaling and see if something comes up for you. I am not kidding, every time I have a physical problem, I seek information from this book and 10/10 times the probable cause is always correct for me.

Listen, I'm not saying to you don't go to a doctor and don't follow modern medicine. Modern medicine absolutely has its value and its place in this world. With that being said, we have been taught for generations that the word of the doctor is gospel and the drugs that they give us are the only answer to our problems. I call bullshit. Disease is a form of dis-ease and for a lot of us our diseases will be caused by a dis-ease mentally.

Think about how your body feels when you are stressed. Maybe you clench your jaw. Maybe your stomach hurts. Maybe you raise your shoulders up towards your ears and tighten them. All of this tension causes constriction and friction in your body and where there is constriction and friction, your body can not function properly. When our body doesn't function properly little issues begin to happen and, over time, they become big issues like TMJ, high blood pressure, irritable bowel syndrome, migraines, etc. In my opinion and in my experience, taking meds, most of the time, especially meds for mental and emotional issues, unless you are clinically diagnosed by a doctor, is like putting a band-aid on a gaping wound that will never heal. And don't even get me started on the side effects. If you truly want to heal or become healthy, you need to do more than just pop a pill. You need to fix whatever is going on mentally and emotionally along with the physical ailment. That is the road to recovery. That is the road to removing dis-ease from your body. The dis-ease is your body telling you there is something deeper than just the ailment that needs to be healed.

I truly don't believe that healing can only be or should only be done through modern medicine. Healing is mind, body, and spirit. There are so many modalities out in the world that you can lean into to help you heal such as acupuncture, chiropractic manipulation, yoga, massage, breathwork, and reiki to name a few.

I live for my chiropractor! I won't lie. I was petrified the first time I went to an appointment at my chiropractor's office. I was experiencing a lot of neck issues along with optical migraines. My dad finally talked me into going. It was some of the best advice he ever gave me. To this day, as long as I visit my chiropractor at least once a month, I don't suffer from the optical migraines. One of the coolest benefits of regularly visiting my chiropractor is that I now have an amazing awareness of my body and I know when I have a subluxation. I also know, depending on where the subluxation is, what may be causing it. For example, if my upper back feels out of whack I can pretty much be sure my allergies or sinuses are out of whack. Then this leads me to look at the seasons to see if my seasonal allergies are raging. If it is not allergy season, then I know it is likely something causing inflammation in my body that will make my sinuses rage. When we have awareness in one area of self it will lead to an awareness in another area of self.

Another healing modality I live for is massage. I try to get a massage once a month and it's not to be bougie. Massages obviously help to reduce stress and increase relaxation. But massages also lessen pain and muscle tightness and increase your immune function. During a massage, toxins are released in your body. That is why it is so important to drink a lot of water after a massage. Our society has put a label on massages as something you do to just relax or something to do to be bougie. There is such a stigma around this healing modality that is intended to relax you as if we are not allowed to relax. We live in a society that is always pushing us to go, go, go. That if we sit down for one second, we are being lazy or selfish. The reality is if we don't take that time for ourselves and take care of our bodies, eventually our bodies are going to make us sit down and we won't have a choice in the matter.

I would have loved to have had someone give me a gift certificate to get a massage when I was a young mom. Carrying around a baby all day long puts a toll on your body, not to mention breast feeding a baby. The positions you can contort your body into so that your baby is comfortable is ridiculous.

The two healing modalities I return to over and over and over again are my meditation and my breathwork. When my meditation practice is consistent, my life just flows like a cool summer breeze. When my meditation practice is not consistent, my life flows like a tornado. My brain is scrambled, my thoughts are darker and more negative, I have a hard time finding positivity in my life, and I don't listen to my intuition. Instead I get too wrapped up in the noise from the outside world. There are so many people these days talking about and teaching meditation, which is fantastic. But just like anything else, the more the chatter about something, the more confusing things become and we start to do things that other people are telling us to do instead of intuitively just following what guides us to what we really need.

Ironically, meditation is something that will help intuitively guide you yet it's hard to find a way to start. What I tell my clients is start small. Start with two minutes. Literally that small. Then when you feel comfortable with two minutes add another minute and so on. Your meditation practice belongs to you. There really is no right or wrong way to meditate and no, you don't need to sit criss-cross applesauce on the floor. If you feel more comfortable in a chair, great. If you feel like lying down, then lie down. Just get comfortable. Maybe sitting isn't your jam when you meditate. Meditation can be achieved through movement. Some people find their running practice their meditation; others find their meditation while they are in the kitchen cooking. Whenever you are in a conscious flow state of being present in the moment focusing on a task that brings you an immense feeling of joy and clarity, that's meditation. This is your meditation practice...do what feels right for you.

The reason we use our breath in a sitting meditation is so that we have a focal point for our thoughts to help them not drift away. I tell my clients to think of their thoughts as clouds in the sky. It's normal for them to be there, because our brains are designed to constantly think, but we don't need to be attached to them. So, while you are sitting in your meditation and thoughts pop up in your head like "I need to wash Cody's baseball pants for his game tomorrow," just notice the thought but not attach to it; let it float by. Attaching to the thought would look like, "I need to wash Cody's baseball pants for his game tomorrow. Oh, and then I need to remind Scott that the girls have soccer practice at 5:30. Crap that means we need to eat dinner early tomorrow. What can I make that is quick and easy?" See how fast your thoughts will just start flowing once you attach yourself to one of them? Then a bunch of thought clouds roll in and before you know it the clouds are storming on your meditation. So, notice the thought and let it float by and then return to your breath. If you need to, count your breath meaning inhale and count to four and then exhale to the count of four. After a few rounds you can release the count.

Breathwork in meditation is a game changer, but it's also a game changer on its own. Whenever I'm feeling anxious or scared or even over-excited, I use breathwork to calm down my nervous system. One form of breathwork that I return to over and over again is what I call 4 x 4. Other people may call it by other names like four squared breath or boxed breath.

HOW TO PRACTICE 4 x 4:

- Inhale through the nose for the count of 4.

- Hold your breath for the count of 4.

- Exhale out of the mouth for the count of 4.

- Hold your breath for the count of 4.

- Repeat for 4 times.

This breathwork can be used during your meditation or you can use this breathwork while you are sitting in traffic and frustrated or standing in a long grocery line on a Sunday morning when there is only one checkout line open. Why do grocery stores do that? You can also use this breathwork when you're standing in front of somebody who is either triggering you or you just aren't interested in what they have to say and you are annoyed. This breathwork is used to calm and regulate your nervous system so it's a great tool to use when you have anxiety.

Another form of breathwork that I like to use I call two-stroke. This breathwork can be used especially when you feel a panic attack coming on. This practice immediately alerts your brain when you take those quick inhales and tells your brain that you want your nervous system to calm down.

HOW TO PRACTICE TWO-STROKE:

- Inhale two fast inhales through the nostrils.

- Exhale a long exhale out your mouth.

- Repeat until you feel your nervous system calm down.

To sum up the emotional self, our emotional self plays a big role in who we are mentally and physically. Taking care of your emotional self daily is crucial in living a healthy and happy life. Our emotions play such a factor in what we believe ourselves to be and the world we live in. Yes, there are outside elements that can determine the trajectory of our lives; however, we have the power within ourselves to decide how we react to those outside elements. We also have the choice to live in a positive mindset or a negative mindset. Those choices can have a huge impact on our physical health and there are so many tools out there to help with our emotions such as therapy, meditation, breathwork, journaling, new thought patterns, and movement. The most important thing I have learned when it comes to emotional self-care is that we should never push down or away our feelings. We need to feel our feelings and sit with them acknowledging them for revealing whatever it is we need to move past in order to move forward. It can be painful and it will suck, but nothing is more painful than being stuck in a feeling forever because you were too scared to release it.

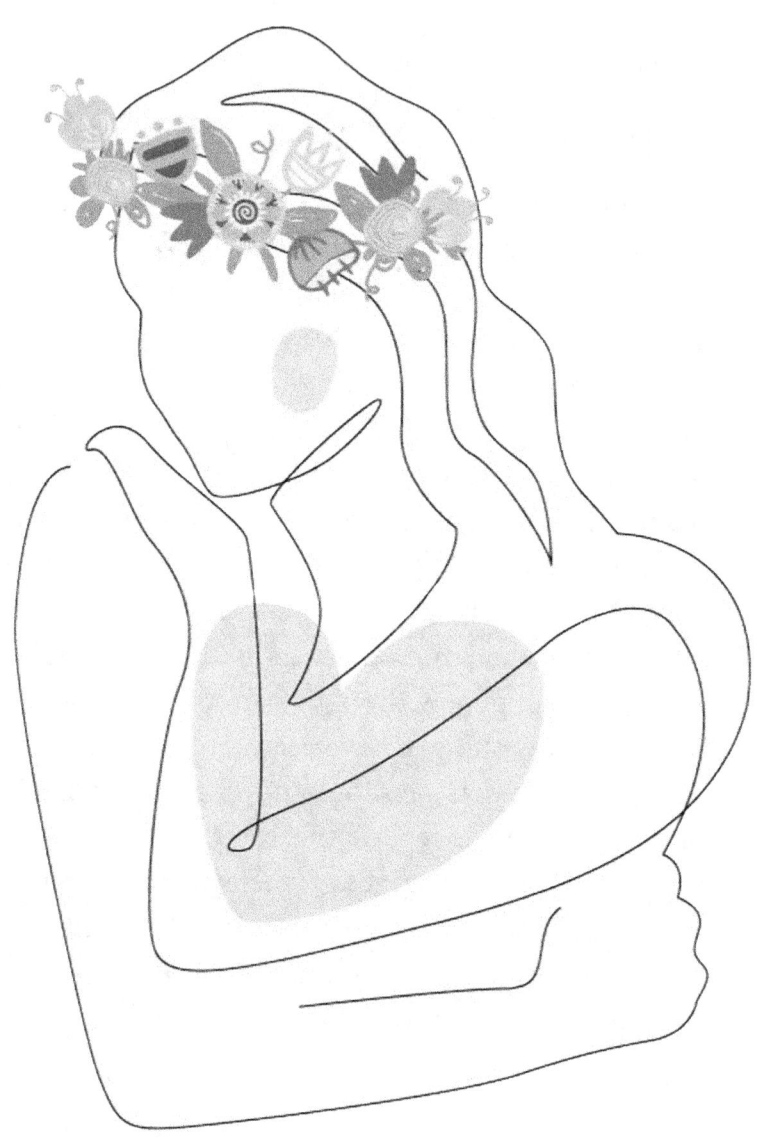

CHAPTER EIGHT

The Intellectual Self

Have you ever heard the phrase, "If you don't use it, you lose it?" That is what happens to your brain, especially as you become older. Intellectual self-care nourishes and challenges your mind. It allows your mind to stay sharp and focused and creative. The more we learn, the more we are able to discuss and communicate with others. We broaden our horizons and have a better understanding of the world we live in.

As children we are constantly learning new things. As our bodies grew, so did our minds. We were being taught all kinds of new knowledge about life, the world, and ourselves. Our brains were constantly being fed in school, but once we graduated from school that constant feeding of the brain slowed down. Sure, maybe we learned something about the job or career we are in, but we sure as hell aren't stimulating our brains the way we used to when we were kids.

In this modern world we don't need to think. Everything is digitally ready to perform tasks for us or just numb our brains out. This is where the hamster wheel comes in. The constant spinning of doing the same thing day in and day out. We aren't challenging ourselves anymore. We aren't learning new and exciting things. Instead we are feeding ourselves the bullshit of social media like Tik Tok and Reels. Look, I love a few minutes of Tik Tok and Reels. They can be fun to watch and yes, you can learn a few things from both of them. However, they were designed to suck you into the blackhole of mind numbing. Be honest. How many times have you clicked on a Reel or Tik Tok and then before you knew it, 20 minutes had passed by? I'm not ashamed to admit it has happened to me, but now I am conscious of it.

There are ways you can battle social media so you do not get sucked into the black hole. Either you can set a certain time out of the day where you allow yourself to look at social media. For example maybe you set a time for 20 minutes in the morning while you sip your coffee or maybe 20 minutes in the evening after you have had dinner. This way you aren't spending multiple times out of the day mindlessly scrolling. You are being intentional about your time. You could also get yourself into the habit of setting a timer every time you click on a social media format so that way you don't accidentally look up from your phone and wonder where your life went.

We need to be conscious about continuously challenging and sharpening our brains. When we keep our brain in tip top shape, we are able to think faster and more clearly. We can process and work through problems, big or small, with more ease. Challenging your brain can be as simple as doing a crossword puzzle or a word find puzzle. Playing games with your family and friends such as board games or card games to challenge your brains can not only be fun, but also can fill up your cup for social self-care. There are plenty of game apps you can play as well with family and friends from a distance.

Challenging our brains also helps with our emotional self-care, not just our intellectual self-care. When we learn about something we enjoy, like a hobby such as photography or baking, we not only are learning and challenging our brains but we also become lit up inside with joy. Researching how to use your camera, what kind of lens you would need, and how to get the lighting right will activate the brain. Think about how your brain feels after a few hours of numbing out on social media or watching Netflix. It's like mush. Now think about how your brain feels after you accomplish a task after doing something you enjoy. You feel energized and you feel happy. Those are the feelings we are striving for to live a healthy and happy lifestyle. I am not telling you to never numb out for 20 minutes on social media or get lost in hours of binge watching Netflix. Sometimes we just need that escape. But if we are using that escape all the time that's a signal something is not right with our emotional self.

When we find something that interests us, we are mostly likely to spend less time scrolling social media mindlessly and laying on the couch or in bed all day binge watching shows. Having a hobby or an interest that requires you to use your brain and challenge your mind helps to keep you focused and sharp. Also having more knowledge about something will pique your interest into other things. For example, when I started to truly practice yoga I began my practice at a local yoga studio strictly for the asana practice. I already had a very consistent workout routine, but I was looking for something to add to my life that would help my body with flexibility and balance. When I left my first yoga class, I got into my car and I needed to sit in park for a few moments. I was so zenned out I was afraid to drive. Once I put my car in drive I drove straight home and pulled into the driveway. I put the car in park and thought, Hmmm, I was supposed to be doing something." Yup I was! I had a list of errands to run including to the grocery store which I drove right past on the way home. Honestly, I was so zen I don't even know how I got home. Between the meditation in the beginning of class and the savasana at the end, I was so freaking relaxed. At that moment I realized I needed more of that feeling in my life. What I thought I needed by going to a yoga class, which was a physical practice, I quickly learned what I needed so desperately was a mindfulness practice.

I realized that I had been practicing mindfulness all of my life. I just wasn't practicing on a consistent basis. Soon after that first yoga class, I was researching and learning about meditation and breathwork. I took classes and workshops to learn techniques on how to meditate to release stress and to deal with, well, life.

I researched breathwork that could help me with anxiety. I am continuously a student, always eager to learn something new. I believe we should constantly learn, especially about the things that light us up, that ignite a fire within us, and that bring us joy.

When we enjoy what we are learning then we are more inclined to put forth effort into that thing. I used this tip when I was teaching writing to my kindergarten and first grade students. Commonly, boys do not enjoy writing. However, when you give them a topic that they enjoy their pencil flows. I had a student one year, who during our writing period, it was like pulling teeth to motivate him to write. He would either just stare at his paper or he would flail around whining that he hated writing.

One day after I was able to get him to refocus through breathwork, I asked him what was one of his most favorite things in the world. Cheeseburgers was his response. So, from that day on for weeks he wrote about nothing but cheeseburgers. To me, at that moment, getting him to somewhat enjoy writing was amazing. I didn't care what the content of the writing was. All I cared about was that he was using the proper strategies I was teaching such as uppercase letters, word spacing, and punctuation. Eventually, I was able to guide him away from writing about cheeseburgers, and he no longer hated writing. That is what happens when you just start with something small. Eventually, it will grow with consistency.

One of the reasons I love reading fiction books so much is because it not only builds our vocabulary, but it allows our minds to wander and be imaginative. As adults we don't allow ourselves the privilege to use our imagination. I do believe it's a privilege to be imaginative. When we read, we create a picture in our minds of what is going on. We know this because when someone makes a movie out of one of our favorite books, most times we don't like the movie as much as the book because it doesn't align with the images we conjured up in our heads.

Why is imagination so important? How do you think things have been created? It starts with a creative thought in the imagination of our minds. When we imagine things, we create things. When we allow our mind to wander our thoughts become ideas. The light bulb, an airplane, the air conditioner that keeps you cool in the summer, these things all began as a thought in someone's mind who was letting their immigration run wild. Reading not only builds our vocabulary and our imagination, but we also learn from reading. Although some fictional books may include fictional places, some books are based on real places and real situations.

Next to reading one of my other favorite modalities to learn from is from listening to a podcast. There are so many podcasts out nowadays, and you can find a podcast to listen to on any subject you may want to learn about or just be entertained by. The podcasts I listen to are podcasts that teach me ways to be a healthier and happier me. Depending on what season of life I am in or what it is I am wanting to learn something about depends on what podcasts I listen to. The top five podcasts I listen to are Divine Downloads, Dear Gabby, Mel Robbins, Jay Shetty, and The Rachel Hollis Podcast. Each of these podcasts always helps me stay on track with my spiritual self-care, but they also double as intellectual self-care. I always learn something on each of those podcasts on how to better myself or connect to my higher power or to help others live a healthy and happy lifestyle.

When I was a teacher, I would mainly listen to podcasts on my daily commute to and from school. Today, I listen to podcasts typically while I am cleaning the house, making dinner, or walking my dogs. I love when a host of a podcast throws out names of books they suggest for their listeners to read on a topic. To me a podcast is like sitting down listening to a good friend talk to me about things that are important to me and giving a good dose of what I need to hear! The podcasts I listen to also often have guests that are experts in areas like health, wellness, mindfulness, and mental health. I get so much juicy information from the guests on the podcasts about information I am truly interested in.

To sum up the intellectual self, if we don't use our brains we begin to lose its power, especially as we age. Challenging our brain and filling it up with knowledge keeps us sharp and focused. With the modern world we live in, especially with the fast pace of technology, we very rarely need to use our brain power to perform a task. Try using one of these tools for intellectual self-care to keep your brain working in tip top shape.

TOOLS FOR INTELLECTUAL SELF-CARE:

- Books
- Research something of interest

- Podcasts

- Games

- Puzzles

- Learn a new hobby

- Take a course on something you enjoy like photography or cooking

CHAPTER NINE

The Spiritual Self

Before I write anything about spiritual self-care, I want to make sure I am very clear on what spirituality is. Spirituality is not about religion, however if your religion ties into your spiritual practice then that's fantastic. You do not have to follow or belong to a religion to be spiritual.

To me, spirituality is your personal relationship to a higher power. You may call that higher power God or Universe. You may have very specific rituals around your higher power such as prayer or meditation or a gratitude practice. Or maybe your spiritual practice is just a very laid back relationship where you speak to your higher power whenever you feel called. For me, my spiritual practice is every day and when I go three or more days without practicing my spiritual habits and rituals, I can begin to find myself in a judgmental and negative spiral.

Spirituality allows us to feel connected to something and in some cases connected to someone. I have what I call my spirit squad. My spirit squad consists of all of my loved ones that have passed on and are now angels, along with my spirit guides, who I have met over the years as I have built my spiritual practice. I also believe that archangels are with me whenever I need them.

I refer to my highest power as God. I was raised Christian and I think, because of that upbringing, I am drawn to calling my higher power God. However, for me God is not a he or a she. God is an energy force that exudes nothing but love. It is my belief that God does not decide the negative things that have happened in our lives nor does God fix them. What I believe God does is exist in a way that shows us that if we lean towards love, even in the darkest of days, we can find light and can find positivity. I think God also is there to remind us that even when something doesn't go the way that we want, we should be grateful for what we do have in our lives. When we lean into that; when we lean into positivity and love no matter what, we will be okay. It doesn't mean life will be easy or without pain, but it does mean that there is infinite possibility of hope.

I have always had a spiritual practice as long as I can remember. I just didn't realize that things like walking barefoot all the time outside, grounding myself to the earth, was a spiritual ritual. I would, as a child and still as an adult, just lay on the ground outside feeling the earth below my body and connecting myself to Mother Earth. My family always found that weird, and to be honest, they still do. Since I was a little girl my parents called me a hippie because I always wanted to be outside barefoot and carefree.

Nature is what I call my church. My favorite church is the coastal line. There is something about sand between my toes and the salty wet air blowing through my hair that soothes my soul. I look out into the ocean and am mesmerized over the idea that there is a whole other world thriving underneath the water. I often wonder if they wonder what it is like up here breathing in the air.

One of the privileges of living in the northeast is that I do get to experience all four seasons and you can bet your ass I take full advantage of that privilege. Each season teaches me valuable lessons in life and each season brings me closer to God. Spring is the time of rebirth and to begin emerging from the hibernation of winter. It's a reminder that we can all start over again at any time. During spring, life begins to pop out and up everywhere you look in nature. The sun starts to shine with longer days than nights. The trees start blooming gorgeous blooms that paint the sky with brilliant colors of pink, and the flowers and plants start emerging from the ground.

Each day you can watch their growth and it's just so fascinating to me that one day I am literally looking at dirt in the ground, and then the next day a little sprout has sprung. Then within weeks a full plant emerges. The grass turns bright green and needs to be cut often filling the air with the smell of freshly cut grass. Baby animals are born and you can see their parents teaching them how to survive in the wild. It truly is a magnificent sight to see. Once spring has sprung and everything has bloomed and the world feels alive people begin to leave their homes more often which means they are moving their bodies more along with eating lighter.

As summer rolls around people continue to be outside more soaking up natural elements like Vitamin D. Mother Nature continues to blossom, vegetable gardens begin to grow, and the heat begins to settle in as people turn to water for recreation. You typically will either find me floating on my raft in my pool or sitting in my beach chair at the Jersey Shore. As the warm summer days slowly turn into chilly fall days, the earth begins to transform again and so do people. The trees begin to change colors and shed their leaves as a sign it is time to let go. The flowers, the plants, and the veggies begin to die off. People begin to start heading back indoors for activities and eating warmer and heavier foods. Before you know it, the trees are bare, the grass is barely green, the gardens are no longer producing and the earth becomes much more still. Animals hibernate and people begin to do the same by spending more time indoors moving their bodies less. This has been my never ending cycle 365 days out of the year for the last 53 years. As much as I absolutely love the summer and would love warm weather all the time, I am grateful for the lessons of new beginnings, growth, letting go, and being still from all of the seasons.

Life is very much like the seasons and what we learn from the seasons is that life is never the same. There are times that are hot and vibrant and full of energy like the summer and there are times that are cold and dark and sluggish like the winter. Each season serves a purpose and so goes the same for the seasons in our life. Without spring new seeds would not be planted so that during the summer those seeds can grow and flourish then be harvested in the fall. Winter allows a break for us to reflect and reorganize our lives if need be. Our spiritual practice can help us during those seasons. Leaning into our spiritual practices allows us to be present in the fun times, reflective in the down times, and grateful even in the hard times.

Like I said, I have always had a spiritual practice, which means I have always had faith in what is happening and what is meant to happen. I also have always had the knowledge that the only way for me to be happy is to make the most out of what my life is right now, even in the shittiest of situations. I also know to accept what is happening in my life no matter what.

As I mentioned earlier, when I was in my late teens, I was extremely sick. It was three years of my life where I literally thought I was dying. I would pray to my God asking for strength to take just one more sip of water as the nurses would hold a cup with a straw next to my hospital bed, because I was too weak to hold the cup myself. There were the times I would lay in the bed and cry. My body ached so bad because I spiked another unexplained high fever. My body was at war and nobody could explain why. Every day I turned to prayer asking God to give me the power and the strength to get through another day. Shit, sometimes it was a prayer to just get through a moment, and every day my God did. Eventually, I was finally on the road to recovery when life smacked me in the face with another winter season.

Since the time I hit puberty at the very young age of 11, I had always had menstruation issues. My doctor wanted to put me on the pill at the age of 13 to regulate my period, but my mom insisted that I was too young. At the time I was pissed because I just didn't want to live with the period pain and the bleeding and the clots, but now that I know what the pill can and does to the body, I am grateful she said no to the pill as my body was developing. Later on, when my mom realized I was having sex, she brought me to the doctor to have him put me on the pill. Her exact words after my doctor asked why I was there for the appointment were, "Well, Christine has decided to start having sex so she needs to go on the pill." That was my mom, very matter of fact, with no concern of how embarrassed I was. Honestly, I loved her for that, even when I was embarrassed. There was no wondering how my mom felt about things or about you. She told you, nice or not.

Unfortunately, as I began to heal from Epstein Barr, I was shortly thereafter diagnosed with endometriosis. I wasn't shocked. My mom had endometriosis and had a full hysterectomy in her early thirties and all of my biological aunts on both sides of my family had hysterectomies in their 40s. What I wasn't expecting to hear after my first surgery to remove the endometriosis is that I would never be able to have children.

I sat in my gynecologist's office in October of 1992 with tears in my eyes as he said to me, "I know you are getting married next year but you need to go home and tell your fiancé that you are not going to be able to have children on your own,

178

and to be honest, I don't think even in vitro will be an option for you." I cried the whole way home and then I cried to my fiancé for hours. Once I settled into the sadness for 24 hours, I sat down with my fiancé and we discussed how we felt about not having children. Up until then, the idea of a family had always been something we both wanted. I didn't want him to regret marrying me because I couldn't give him a child. He asked me how I felt about not being able to have children. At that moment I felt a wave rush over me and I said, "I want us to be able to have children, but that moment isn't even something we are considering right now. I think that when the time comes for us to build a family what is meant to happen will. Maybe we adopt or maybe we use a surrogate? Who knows. I think for right now we focus on getting married and then when we decide about building a family later." He was absolutely on board with that conversation.

We continued with the preparations for the wedding in August of 1993 and had everything set for our wedding from my dress to the church to the venue to the photographer. In February of 1993, I noticed my jeans were getting tight over my hips. Even though I didn't think it was possible for me to become pregnant, a little voice inside my head kept whispering to take a pregnancy test. There they were, two lines. It was positive. Scott and I were so fucking happy, nervous, but happy. My mom jumped up and hugged me and started to cry when I told her and she whispered in my ear, "I'm so happy for you. I didn't think this was ever going to happen." Quickly I began making phone calls to change our wedding date. This is why I know God exists. Every single place that we had booked for

August was opened on the date in May of 1993 we wanted to get married. It was all divine timing. In October of 1993, one year later from the time I was told I wouldn't have children, I was holding my son in my arms.

That's the thing about spiritual practice. When we learn to let go of our expectations of what we think is supposed to happen in life, and we lean into love and acceptance of what is happening in life at this moment, then what is supposed to happen will unfold in divine timing, as it should. I let go of the vision of what I thought building my family would look like. I allowed loving thoughts and acceptance into my life instead of bitterness and control over the situation, and I was blessed with not one, but three beautiful and amazing children who are fucking amazing adults that I couldn't be more proud of today. I absolutely believe my surrender to the acceptance of the possibility of not having a family allowed me to relax and allowed my body to heal so that I could become pregnant.

Becoming pregnant wasn't the only time I had to lean into my spiritual practice when it came to my children. I have had to lean into my spiritual practice a lot as a mom. One of the most difficult times was when not one of my daughters, but both of my daughters, were born premature and spent time in NICU.

First, let me just say that NICU nurses and doctors are angels on earth. After each delivery they saved my daughters' lives, and I will forever be in gratitude to them and in awe of them. I would lean into my spiritual practice asking for strength and guidance to be the best mama I could be in those moments. Nothing prepares you to see your child hooked up to machines with tubes running down their throat and monitors all over their body. I'll never forget the feeling in the pit of my stomach, actually I can feel it right now, when I think about the time the nurse called me at home and said, "Your daughter's veins keep collapsing, so when you come in she may have an IV on her scalp."

We were lucky and fortunate, both girls left the NICU with no complications or needing any more medical assistance. The entire time they spent in NICU, I would tap into my spirit squad for them to protect them. I would lean into faith and believe that they would be okay. I would talk to God many times throughout the day. I also sat in gratitude every day after watching each of my daughters during their stay in NICU as they got a little bit stronger every day, and I expressed my heartfelt gratitude to the staff for their hard work and effort.

A gratitude practice allows us to find the good in our lives. I have had a daily ritual of writing a gratitude practice for years now. Each day I write at least three things I am grateful for that have happened in the last 24-48 hours. The reason I write about something that has happened within the last 24-48 hours is because we can all write a broad statement such as, "I am grateful for my family." But what exactly are you grateful for? When we look for specific things to be grateful for, like "I am grateful that I woke up today in a beachfront hotel in Florida with my husband, because we both deserve and needed a much needed brain reset. It was amazing to roll out of bed and stand on the balcony and look out into the ocean through the palm trees and exhale," gratitude has more meaning to it.

When we find specific moments in our gratitude practice that we can write about, we are more inclined throughout the day to notice all the positive little things that are happening in our lives. We might catch something out of the corner of the eye and pause to enjoy it instead of barreling through our day just checking off our to-do list.

Gratitude changes our mindset from a lack mentality to an abundant mentality. The more you find gratitude in things the more things for you to be grateful for will appear in your life because you will now notice them. Have you ever noticed if you are looking to purchase something like a specific model car and once you decide that is the model of the car you are going to buy, you then see that model of car everywhere? That is exactly what happens when you choose gratitude. You will begin to constantly see the things in you that make you grateful because those things are always there. You just need to be willing and wanting to see them.

This next part of my spiritual practice may not resonate with some of you, but I feel I need to be my authentic self and share it with you. If this doesn't resonate with you, no worries! Your spiritual practice is your spiritual practice and you do you. I, however, would like for you to read this with an open mind, because you never know when something that may have never resonated with you one day may actually resonate with you at a different season of life.

As I mentioned before I have a spiritual squad. I believe that I have angels and guides and archangels with me at all times. I believe they are here to guide me and support me and protect me through life. When I am consistent with my self-care practice, especially my spiritual self, my mind, body, and spirit are aligned. I can feel my spirit squad presence all the time. When I meditate, I call in my spiritual squad to help guide my meditations. When I am receiving energy healing, I can feel their presence in the room and I know they are helping my energy healer heal me. I know this, because she tells me when they speak to her as well and she relays their messages to her with me. Whenever I meet with a psychic or medium, they always comment that my angels are present, and then usually follow that up by saying there are a lot of them and they talk a lot and over top one another. This always makes me giggle, because that is how I see and hear my spirit squad. I love them so much.

The first time I was approached by an angel it was my uncle. He passed away in 1988 in his early 30s to lymphoma. He left behind my aunt and their two kids, a daughter and a son. After his passing, my aunt and cousins moved into my parent's house with us. I loved my uncle. He was one of my favorite people. He was always playing games with people and making everyone laugh so hard, including me.

One night shortly after my aunt and cousins moved in, my uncle came to me in a dream. I will never forget the image. He was sitting in our rocking chair in the living room with a yellow polo shirt on and khakis. His left leg was extended further than the right and he was rocking the chair with his right foot flat on the floor. He was smiling at me and told me how he missed everyone. Then he told me he needed me to do him a favor and asked me if I would watch over my cousin, his daughter. "She's a tough one to crack," he said. "And she's going to need someone to lean on." With tears in my eyes, I without hesitation said yes and to this day I have continued to do him that favor.

His daughter, my cousin, is one of the best friends I have had in my life. Even though we are eight years apart, we have grown up together and raised our babies together. Our husbands are best of friends and we vacation with one another. I sometimes wonder if me doing him a favor was actually him doing me a favor, because my cousin is one of the most important persons in my life. Since that first encounter with my uncle, I have had so many encounters with him and many other angels of mine that I have lost count. I love my interactions with my angels. They remind me that even when we lose someone from their vessel (their body) we don't ever actually lose them. Like my Gram taught me at her father's funeral, as long as we keep them in our mind and in our heart, they are never gone.

My angels don't always come in the form of humans. Sometimes they show up as a butterfly or a dime or a feather or an animal. Sometimes I will call on my angels and ask them to come to me in a certain form, especially when I need guidance or I just need to not feel like I am alone. Most of the time, they just show up on their own. When I am truly aligned in mind, body and spirit my angels are dropping signs left and right. When I am not aligned in mind, body, and spirit, then I barely see them. Don't worry. They are still there. It's just that I have my head so wrapped up in bullshit that I don't have the awareness they are even there.

When we are aligned, we become very in tune with the guidance that our angels give us. Our angels are there to help guide us into making good life choices. You know that gut feeling you get when you are trying to decide something or something seems not right? That is your angel signaling to you caution! You know that inner voice you hear from time to time that actually has a dialogue inside your brain? Those are your angels talking to you. Listen up!

When I practice my spiritual self-care, there are certain tools that I like to use during my rituals. One item is burning palo santo. I use palo santo every day to clear out negative energy and promote positivity from myself and my house. You could also use sage. I personally am not a fan of the smell of sage, but if I need some heavy duty clearing, I will use sage. But palo santo is my fav and my number one go to! I also like to light palo santo before I meditate to clear my space and my mind. Do I think palo santo has some magical dust inside of it? No. I do believe that ritual along with the smell and the embers lit while the smoke leaves the stick evokes a calmness within me because it contains the constituent d-limonene. This oil is very therapeutic to the emotions and balances the root chakra. The ritual of burning palo santo has been around for centuries in many cultures and it continues to be carried on from generation to generation.

Another tool I like to use during my spiritual self-care practice is crystals. Just like palo santo, the use of crystals for rituals has been around for many centuries. Depending on which chakra (or area of the body) I would like some extra loving and healing around, I use crystals to send energy to those areas. For example, if I want more self-love, I will carry around rose quartz.

Rose quartz is a stone of both giving and receiving love. When my reiki clients are blocked in their heart chakras, I often advise them to purchase rose quartz. Crystals can be carried in your pocket or bra (don't forget to remove them before you put them in the hamper!) or purse to carry them around with you. You can also place them on your nightstand to emit energy while you sleep or place the crystal on your desk while you work or somewhere in your car. I personally like to purchase pieces of jewelry such as a necklace, earrings, or bracelets with the crystals in them. Wearing them as a piece of jewelry makes it easier to have them in my possession at all times.

I not only wear or carry my crystals, I use them as a ritual during my meditation. Depending on what I want to manifest in my life or an area of my life or personal self I need healing, I will hold the crystal in my left hand during my meditation. Why the left hand? The left hand is the receiving hand as the right hand is the giving hand. When you want to resonate with the crystal's energy or absorb healing energies through your body during your meditation, you would want to hold the crystal in your left hand. You would also wear your crystal bracelet on the left wrist for the same reason. When you want to release toxins and negative energies or manifest your intentions you would want to hold your crystal in your right hand or wear your crystal bracelet on your right wrist.

Another tool I use in my spiritual practice is oracle cards. Oracle cards are designed to help reveal to you the present energy you are projecting, but to also reveal the result you are likely to attract. There are many different types of oracle cards from spirit animals to female goddesses to angels to affirmations to sacred symbols, the list runs the gamut. I recommend to my clients when choosing what type of oracle cards they would like to use to go with their gut instinct at the moment and grab a deck. If you are unsure which deck to choose, take a moment to center yourself and take a deep inhale and long exhale, and ask your angels, guides, and your highest power to guide you to what you need at the moment.

When purchasing cards, just go with whatever resonates the most with you, whether it's just a gut feeling or the cover of deck is aesthetically pleasing to you. I have many types of oracle cards, but my favorite type of oracle cards are affirmation cards. I choose one affirmation card at random daily in the morning and I use that affirmation throughout the day. I also choose a deck of cards prior to meditations, and before my meditation I will pull a card. If I want to be guided through my meditation, I will look at my card. If I do not want guidance from my card during my meditation, I will look at the card after the meditation. Most times than not the card will reference something that came through in my meditation.

Using these tools during my spiritual practice helps me to feel more grounded and connected to myself and my higher power. Being connected to something does not mean you need to be able to see it. We all experience love but we don't see it. We may see acts of love like a hug or a kiss but there is nothing visible about love. It is a feeling. It is knowing that it exists. Spirituality is the ultimate essence of love. It's surrendering to the unknown with unwavering faith and trust knowing that you are being guided to not only where you belong in the future but also knowing you are exactly where you belong now, regardless of if it's a hard season or an easy season.

Spirituality is also the greatest teacher because when we practice spiritual self-care, we find the awareness of our flaws and our mistakes and we honor them and accept them. We learn from them. Having faith in the unknown gives you a superpower of faith within yourself. When you surrender to a power greater than yourself you surrender your ego allowing your authentic truth to come forward. When you are your authentic self with no hesitation of showing the world who you are, you can be an unstoppable beam of light shining in this world.

My greatest tool for my spiritual practice is meditation. I have spoken already about meditation a few chapters back. Meditation is a tool that can be used for so many parts of self, but if you truly want to find connection with the divine, to call in your highest power, guides, and angels then meditation is THE tool to practice. I often say to my clients, prayer is when we speak to God but meditation is when we listen to God. Whether our meditation is in stillness or in movement, when we find ourselves in a flow state where our thoughts are flowing like a river, we begin to hear answers to questions we have been longing to hear. We might not like the answers we may hear, but the answers are always the answers that are for our highest good. I recommend to my clients to try to meditate for at least 10 minutes a day. However, I understand that some days are crazier than others. Even if you have only two minutes a day, close your eyes and focus on a few long inhales and long exhales.

To sum up the spiritual self, spirituality is our hope, our faith, and our belief system. When we have a spiritual self-care practice we learn to live through life with gratitude, with ease and with grace no matter how good or bad our life is at the moment. We have faith and hope that we will find the strength to get us through anything that may come our way. We also have the ability to be present in the moment enjoying all the wonderful moments that come our way. A spiritual self-care practice is a daily reminder that we are all one and our only mission in life is to love and to be loved by others and by our Self.

Tools for spiritual practice:

Gratitude list: Write three things you are grateful for that have happened in the last 24-48 hours and write why you are grateful for them.

Ask for a sign: When you are looking for guidance from the universe that you are not alone or that you are being guided in the right direction ask for a sign to be delivered to you.

Palo Santo: Burn palo santo as a ritual to clear out negative energy and to evoke positive energy around yourself or a room or your entire house.

Crystals: Carry or wear crystals that resonate with the area you would like healing or would like to manifest.

Oracle cards: Choose a deck of cards that resonate with you. Pulling a card can be done at any point of the day and can be used as a ritual before a practice such as meditation.

Meditation: Meditate for 10 minutes a day.

CHAPTER TEN

Habit Stacking
(The Secret to Creating a Daily Self-Care Practice)

So how do we create a daily self-care practice? Pick an area of self: physical, social, emotional, intellectual, or spiritual that you would like to focus on. Then pick a habit or ritual that you would like to create for that area that will leave you feeling healthy and happy. Practice that habit or ritual for 21 days. Continue with that habit or ritual and then stack a new habit or ritual for either that same area or a new area for another 21 days, and so on. Creating a self-care practice takes time. I recommend trying one habit or ritual at a time but you know yourself better than anyone else. If you think you can handle two habits at a time, go for it! In fifteen weeks, you should have a solid foundation for your daily self-care practice that is mind, body, and spirit aligned.

Consistency is the key to a successful daily self-care practice and keeping yourself aligned, mind, body, and spirit. When you are consistent your days will flow with a lot more ease, you will be able to manage your thoughts and emotions better, and when shit hits the fan, when the storm rolls in, you are equipped with enough tools to weather the storm. Will you slip from time to time? Of course. You are human. I do it all the time. What I have come to find though is that I have a magic number. It is 3. If I go beyond 3 days of not practicing my habits and rituals for the five areas of self, I know that I will have a harder time getting back on track of them. The longer you go without doing your practice, the harder it becomes to get back into the habit.

If I know I am going on a vacation, I am very intentional that the few days before I come home I start gearing myself up with pep talks of the things I need to return to when I arrive home, which typically is my physical practice around eating healthier and working out. Depending on the type of vacation, I may also fall off of my spiritual practice as well. I also am so self aware now from having had a daily self-care practice for years that I know when I am feeling or acting a certain way due to not practicing a habit or ritual. When I feel myself feeling agitated easily, I know that I have not been free flow journaling. For me, I need to get my thoughts and emotions out on the page everyday to sort them out or release them.

I also want for you to be aware that as seasons change, so will your habits and rituals. Do not feel that because you were doing something five years ago that you need to be doing that same thing now. You are not the same person you were five years ago. So if you feel that what you are practicing just isn't resonating with you, then try tweaking it, adding to it, or just drop it and try something else.

***

What I have shared in this book are all the tips and tools that I have learned to shape and create my own daily self-care practice. Just because I practice a certain habit or ritual absolutely does not mean you need to do the same. The only thing I highly recommend when creating your daily self-care practice that is the same is to create a habit or ritual that focuses on each of the five areas of self and practice them daily.

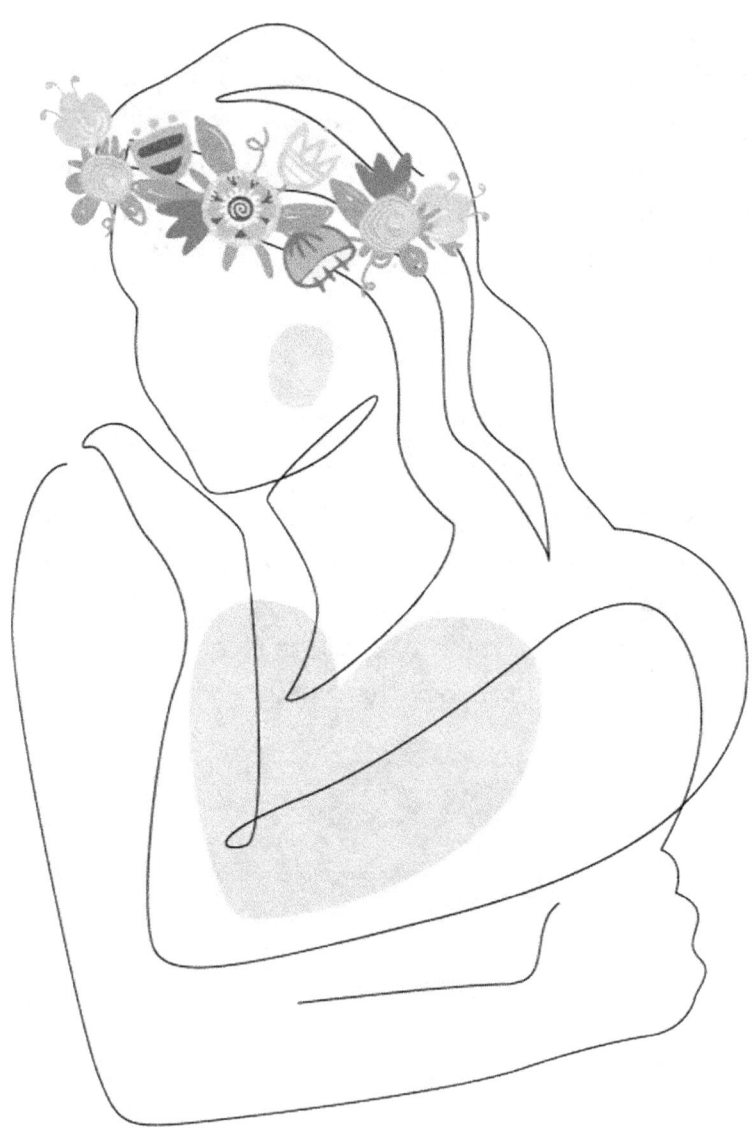

CHAPTER ELEVEN

Create Your Own Daily Self-Care Practice

It's now time to begin to create your own daily self-care practice. Under each area of self, I have three suggestions of habits and rituals that you can choose from to begin creating your daily self-care practice. As I stated before, this is your daily self-care practice. If something does not resonate with you, then choose something of your own that does and will be aligned with that area of self.

After you choose a habit or ritual, answer the question of

why you want to incorporate this habit or ritual. For example, maybe under physical self-care you write, "I will eat healthier foods, because I am pre-diabetic and I do not want to become a Type 2 diabetic. Or maybe under social self-care you write, "I will make a date with a friend once a week, because I miss seeing and talking to my friends. I need that interaction in my life to make me happy." When we attach a reason why to something we are going to do it gives that something a purpose and a meaning, instead of just thinking you might want to do something.

PHYSICAL SELF-CARE

- Choose a movement you enjoy and do that for 30 minutes a day. Don't choose running if you hate running! Pick something you ENJOY! And here's a hack: try 15 minutes in the morning and 15 minutes in the evening.

- Drink half your weight in ounces of water daily. Try using a measured water bottle or put a hydration app on your phone.

- Get 6-8 hours of sleep at night. Begin by creating a bedtime ritual or try to go to bed 30 minutes earlier.

Write which habit or ritual you would like to begin incorporating into your daily self-care practice and why:

_____

_____

_____

_____

_____

SOCIAL SELF-CARE

- Make a weekly or monthly date day or dinner with your friends.

- Talk to two people in your circle every day through text, phone calls, Snapchat, or in person.

- Plan weekly or monthly family dinners.

Write which habit or ritual you would like to begin incorporating into your daily self-care practice and why:

_____

_____

_____

_____

EMOTIONAL SELF-CARE

- Meditate daily even if you only have 5 minutes.

- Free flow journal: write whatever thoughts you are having for 3 pages daily in your journal

- Set a boundary with a person, place, or thing.

Write which habit or ritual you would like to begin incorporating into your daily self-care practice and why:

_____

_____

_____

_____

_____

INTELLECTUAL SELF-CARE

- Listen to podcasts while driving, cleaning, or working out.

- Read a book for at least 15 minutes a day. Do this before you go to bed or stop taking your phone in the bathroom and take a book instead.

- Play card games or board games with a friend or even a game on an app, and invite friends to play along.

Write which habit or ritual you would like to begin incorporating into your daily self-care practice and why:

_____

_____

_____

_____

SPIRITUAL SELF-CARE

- Write a daily gratitude list of 3-5 things you are grateful for that has happened in the last 24-48 hours.

- Pray daily.

- Go outside in nature as much as possible. Nature provides healing energy.

Write below which habit or ritual you would like to begin incorporating into your daily self-care practice and why:

_____

_____

_____

_____

_____

On the following pages you will find a quick and easy "Habit Tracker" to track your progress each day. Seeing your progress written down gives you the visual confirmation of how well you are doing, or it could have the complete opposite effect of letting you know where you need help. If you find that you chose a habit or ritual and you notice that you are not staying consistent with it, then reevaluate that habit or ritual. It may not be the right habit or ritual for you, and that is okay. Give yourself grace! This is a journey not a destination. It will take time and it will take some learning along the way.

If there is anything I would like for you to take away from reading this book, and thank you by the way for reading this book because by reading this book you are working on trying to be the best version of yourself. I want you to remember this, you are completely in control of your health and happiness. The choices you make on how you live your life and how you choose to let people exist in your life will dictate your health and happiness. Choose you, along with everyone else. You matter. So go ahead and be me-ish!

HABIT TRACKER

AREA OF SELF: _____

HABIT/RITUAL	M	T	W	T	F	S	S
1.							
2.							
3.							
4.							
5.							
6.							
7.							
8.							
9.							
10.							

HABIT/RITUAL	M	T	W	T	F	S	S
11.							
12.							
13.							
14.							
15.							
16.							
17.							
18.							
19.							
20.							
21.							

Acknowledgments

The words in this book would not be possible without the deep life lessons you taught me Mommy. I am forever grateful to be your daughter. I wish you were here to read these pages. I promise not to bend my pages when I read them.

Scott, Cody, Casey, Kylie, Sabrina, Adam, Mike, Christopher, Cayden, and grandbaby on the way. You are the light of my life. The breath in my lungs. You are the reason I reach for the best version of me so that I can be my best version for you. You are the purpose behind my passion for A Healthy and Happy You. I love you with all of my heart.

Daddy, thank you for always being my rock, my biggest supporter, and keeping me sane in this crazy thing called life.

Cassandra Bodzak; my mentor, writing coach, spiritual guru, and friend. Thank you for being the catalyst for this book. It has been years in the making and I am grateful you have been with me every step of the way guiding me with everything that is practical and magical.

Fay Thompson you have been the missing piece to the puzzle for putting this book together. Thank you for your creative insight and your patience. I could not have done it without you.

My students and clients, you are my guiding light. I am so very thankful for your trust in me to guide you through your journey to a healthy and happy you.

About the Author

CHRISSY KOHUT is the owner and founder of **A Healthy and Happy You,** a wellness studio located in New Jersey, where she coaches and teaches her clients how to live a healthy and happy lifestyle through mindfulness and self-care practices.

Chrissy, a former elementary school teacher, is a self-care specialist, a certified yoga instructor for adults and children, and a Reiki practitioner. She offers yoga classes, Reiki sessions, and self-care workshops online and at her studio.

Chrissy enjoys helping her clients and students by sharing all the tips and tools she has learned along the way from her teachers, coaches, mentors, and from her own life experiences as a wife of over thirty years, a mother to three grown children, and two grandsons. Chrissy's motto is: "It's a good day to have a good day," and truly believes that with a positive mindset and a daily self-care practice, it is possible to be a "A Healthy and Happy You."

To learn more about Chrissy and her work visit:

 www.ahealthyandhappyyou.com

 Instagram@ahealthyandhappyyou